NATIONAL INSTI
SERVICES L

Volume 2

CARING FOR PEOPLE

CARING FOR PEOPLE
Staffing Residential Homes

NATIONAL COUNCIL OF
SOCIAL SERVICE

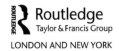

Routledge
Taylor & Francis Group
LONDON AND NEW YORK

First published in 1967 by George Allen & Unwin Ltd

This edition first published in 2022
by Routledge
4 Park Square, Milton Park, Abingdon, Oxon OX14 4RN
605 Third Avenue, New York, NY 10017

Routledge is an imprint of the Taylor & Francis Group, an informa business

© 1967 by Taylor & Francis.

British Library Cataloguing in Publication Data
A catalogue record for this book is available from the British Library

ISBN: 978-1-03-203381-5 (Set)
ISBN: 978-1-00-321681-0 (Set) (ebk)
ISBN: 978-1-03-206914-2 (Volume 2) (hbk)
ISBN: 978-1-03-206926-5 (Volume 2) (pbk)
ISBN: 978-1-00-320458-9 (Volume 2) (ebk)

DOI: 10.4324/9781003204589

Publisher's Note
The publisher has gone to great lengths to ensure the quality of this reprint but points out that some imperfections in the original copies may be apparent.

Disclaimer
The publisher has made every effort to trace copyright holders and would welcome correspondence from those they have been unable to trace.

CARING FOR PEOPLE

STAFFING RESIDENTIAL HOMES

THE REPORT OF
THE COMMITTEE OF ENQUIRY
SET UP BY THE
NATIONAL COUNCIL OF SOCIAL SERVICE

Chairman

GERTRUDE WILLIAMS
C.B.E.

London
GEORGE ALLEN & UNWIN LTD
RUSKIN HOUSE MUSEUM STREET

FIRST PUBLISHED IN 1967
SECOND IMPRESSION 1968

© *George Allen & Unwin Ltd 1967*

SBN 04 360015 8

PRINTED IN GREAT BRITAIN

*in 11 on 12 point Fournier type
by C. Tinling & Co. Ltd.
Liverpool, London & Prescot*

MEMBERSHIP OF COMMITTEE

CHAIRMAN
>Professor Lady Williams, C.B.E.
>*Emeritus Professor of Social Economics*
>*University of London*

‡Dr Mark Abrams
Chairman, Research Services Ltd

Mr R. H. Adams
formerly Principal, Kingswood Schools, Bristol

§Miss Mary Applebey, O.B.E.
General Secretary, National Association for Mental Health

§Miss G. M. Aves, C.B.E.
formerly Chief Welfare Officer, Ministry of Health

‡Miss E. F. F. Blencowe, S.R.N.
Matron-in-Charge, Hastings House, Loughborough

*‡Rev Andrew J. Buchan
Secretary and Director, Church of Scotland Social and Moral Welfare Board

§Miss S. Clement Brown, O.B.E.
National Institute for Social Work Training, formerly Director of Child Care Studies, Home Office Children's Department

Mr George Evans, O.B.E.
County Welfare Officer, Cheshire County Council

§‡Dr J. M. Gibbs, O.B.E.
Lecturer in Psychology, University College, Cardiff

Mr J. Hanson
Chief Welfare Officer, London Borough of Bromley

§Mr R. Huws Jones, *Vice-Chairman*
Principal, National Institute for Social Work Training

Sir Herbert Pollard, C.B.E.
formerly Treasurer, City and County of Kingston-upon-Hull

Dr Elisabeth Shoenberg
Consultant Psychiatrist, Claybury Hospital and London Hospital M.R.C. Social Medicine Research Unit

‡Mr T. F. Tucker, O.B.E.
formerly General Superintendent, Dr Barnado's Homes

§‡Miss S. Watson, O.B.E.
County Children's Officer, Hertfordshire County Council

†Professor Roger Wilson
Professor of Education and Social Development, University of Bristol

ASSESSOR
Sir George Haynes, C.B.E.
Director, National Council of Social Service

SECRETARY: Mrs M. A. Ogilvy-Webb

ADVISORS:
The following Government Departments and other organizations appointed official Advisors to the Committee:

Department of Education and Science
Ministry of Health
Home Office
Scottish Education Department
Scottish Home and Health Department
Ministry of Health and Social Services, N. Ireland
Northern Ireland Council of Social Service.

---

* Mr Buchan died in July 1965.
† Professor Wilson resigned in January 1966 on taking up a prolonged visiting appointment in the University of Malawi.
‡ Member of Census Sub-Committee.
§ Member of Training Sub-Committee.

CONTENTS

FOREWORD

by Sir George Haynes

The demand for the enquiry on which this report is based came from workers in the field of residential care, both those in voluntary organizations and those in Local Authorities, who were responsible for staffing residential establishments. They felt growing concern on account of the present shortage of staff, the constantly increasing complexity of the work to be done and the realization that these problems are likely to be even more serious in the future than they are now.

The National Council of Social Service was therefore asked to promote an investigation into the staffing of residential establishments to cover the whole field of residential care. The Council agreed to do this and received a generous grant for the purpose from the Calouste Gulbenkian Foundation.

The Committee was appointed in October 1962 with the following terms of reference:

'To enquire into the recruitment and retention, training and field of work of the staff of residential accommodation, other than hospitals, designed for persons in need of care, whether short or long term, and whether provided by statutory authorities, voluntary bodies or otherwise, and to make recommendations.'

It was decided that the detailed consideration of salaries, which are the responsibility of many different negotiating bodies, should be excluded, but the broad principles were discussed and are referred to in the Report, especially in Chapter 6 and in recommendations 12-14 at the end of that chapter.

The Council was fortunate in enlisting a Committee, under the chairmanship of Professor Lady Williams, whose combined knowledge and experience have been of incalculable value. It should be stressed that the members were invited to act as individual experts and not as representatives of any organization with which they are connected; but between them they covered the whole field with which the enquiry was concerned. The Council also invited the appropriate Government Departments to nominate observers to assist the Committee in their discussions.

The National Council of Social Service would like to place on record their appreciation of the contribution made by Lady Williams, the members of the Committee and the observers. The knowledge, enthusiasm and sheer hard work which they brought to their task can only be fully appreciated by those who were privileged to share in their discussions. In particular their thanks are due to the Chairman, Lady Williams, who, in addition to the heavy burden of leading the discussion in the very numerous and lengthy meetings, undertook the major work of writing the greater part of the Report in its final form.

During the course of the Committee's discussions it became clear that two topics of great importance would need to be worked out in considerable detail. The first was the need to collect factual information about the staffs working in residential institutions; the second was concerned with training. Two sub-committees were therefore set up.

The first, under the chairmanship of Dr Mark Abrams was responsible for drawing up the questionnaire and arranged for the two pilot surveys to test it.

The second, under the chairmanship of Dr John Gibbs, gave detailed consideration to the whole problem of training for residential care and drafted the form and content of the training recommendations.

The Council is grateful for the immense amount of work and the expert knowledge contributed by these two sub-committees.

This Report is the product of the deliberations of devoted people who have worked hard and long. It is designed for use. The Council commends it for action to government departments, local authorities, voluntary organizations and all those who are concerned with the welfare of old people, children and adults in residential care now, or who will be in the future.

CHAIRMAN'S PREFACE

I am glad to have an opportunity of putting on record my thanks to the many people who have helped in this Enquiry. First and foremost my thanks go to the members of the Committee. Their names are evidence of the wide range of knowledge and experience on which we could call but, in addition, they have worked tirelessly throughout the four years that the task has taken. No Chairman could hope for a more cooperative and congenial group of colleagues.

A sad note was struck by the tragic death of the Reverend Andrew J. Buchan which took place actually during one of our weekend conferences. We all mourned the loss of a friend. His contribution to our discussions had been of great value and his death deprived us of his wise counsel. The Reverend L. Beattie Garden of the Church of Scotland Social and Moral Welfare Board was invited to take his place on the Committee but Mr Beattie Garden felt that he could give us little assistance at such a late stage in our proceedings. All papers were sent to him so that he could make any comments he wished to have considered, but he did not attend any meetings and so does not sign the Report.

Next our thanks must go to our observers and, in particular, to Mr S. A. Gwynn of the Home Office, Mr J. E. Pater of the Ministry of Health and Mr I. M. Wilson of the Scottish Education Department, all of whom devoted a great deal of attention to the Enquiry and helped us with their detailed knowledge.

We owe much to the local authorities and to the national committees of the large voluntary organizations without whose help we should have found it impossible to distribute and to collect the questionnaires which provide the statistical basis of our Enquiry. Their readiness to cooperate stemmed from their own anxiety with regard to the subject of our investigation but they gave their help unstintingly. We are very grateful to them.

We are grateful, too, to the many organizations and individuals who prepared written memoranda for our consideration and to the large number of people who came to give oral evidence to us. A list appears in Appendix A.

It is customary for Committees of Enquiry to express their thanks to their secretary but, in our case, the tribute we wish to offer is no mere form of words. Throughout our task we have had the help, as Research and Organizing Secretary, of Mrs Marjorie Ogilvy-Webb. Her mastery of the subject, her ability to summarize detailed evidence, her organizing capacity and her personal qualities have made a major contribution to our work. It proved impossible to do as we had hoped and provide her with a Deputy secretary to help her in this work, for both those appointed were compelled to give up after a short time for health or domestic reasons; and this difficulty accounts, in part, for the fact that the Enquiry has taken rather longer than was first intended. But fortunately Mrs Ogilvy-Webb had the assistance of a very small, but hard-working and loyal, office staff particularly Mrs Parsons-Smith to whom also our thanks are due.

The Report is, therefore, very much the result of cooperative effort and all who have played a part in it hope that it will be given urgent and serious consideration by those who have it in their power to further the welfare of the men, women and children in residential care.

GERTRUDE WILLIAMS

1

THE PROBLEM BEFORE US

1. During recent years there has been a growing volume of disquiet over the difficulty of staffing the residential Homes which care for the thousands of men, women and children who, for one reason or another, cannot be cared for in their own homes. Representations have been made from many quarters that a comprehensive enquiry was called for which might lead to constructive suggestions for a radical improvement in the situation.

2. One of the most important social tasks is carried out by those entrusted with the care of these people living in institutions of one kind or another. The pressure on existing accommodation is already very great and we believe (and give our reasons for this belief in a later chapter) that the demand is likely to increase.

3. In view of the present social policy, which emphasizes the value of facilities which enable people in need of help to remain in their own homes whenever possible, it may be asked why there should be any great need for residential care, either now or in the future. The question is very pertinent, because the reasons why people cannot remain in their own homes throw light on the problems of those who care for them in residential establishments.

4. Much has been done, for example, to expand the domiciliary services, both statutory and voluntary, to help elderly men and women to live with their families or on their own; home helps, meals on wheels, specially designed housing, home equipment adapted to the needs of the old, chiropody services and so on. Nevertheless, there are many whose needs cannot be met in this way. With increasing old age (and many more now live to a ripe old age) they become increasingly infirm and can no longer manage the shopping and housework, or they require assistance with dressing or must spend occasional days in bed. In many such cases a daughter or niece living near by can provide all the assistance needed, or a kindly neighbour undertakes the simple duties required. But with the growing amount of personal mobility,

the younger members of the family move to housing estates or to the New Towns or to another locality where better work is available, and this leaves a growing number of older people who have no relations living near enough to help in these ways. We are so accustomed to thinking of people as members of family groups that it is sometimes difficult to remember that very many have no kith and kin. According to Professor Townsend's study of old people living in residential Homes, 40 per cent had never been married, and 59 per cent had no surviving children[1]. In many instances, even where there are members of the family in the neighbourhood, there is not enough room in the flat or house to provide accommodation for an older person whose health calls for a room to himself, or who finds the strain of living in the midst of a healthy noisy younger group too much for him; and advancing age increases the difficulty. The elderly who need residential care are therefore very much older than used to be the case before so much domiciliary assistance was provided; and many of them are infirm or confused. This involves a different kind of care from that needed by those who are younger and healthier.

5.   A similar change in the nature of the need is found in other groups. Increasingly, the social services are supporting and helping incomplete and inadequate families so that children do not have to be removed from their homes because of poverty or neglect or lack of care. Sometimes, however, family break-up cannot be prevented or children may need help, guidance and training which cannot be provided in their own homes. Some may need special schooling because of severe physical or mental handicap for which day provision cannot be made. Sometimes, children may need a temporary refuge whilst mother is in hospital or during some other family catastrophe. The tendency today is to place children who have to leave their natural home in foster-homes, but some among them are so difficult in their behaviour or so emotionally disturbed as a result of their life experience that they need skilled, remedial care. Few foster-homes can give such children the help which they need and they are placed in residential establishments. To care for such children and to work with their parents makes different demands on the staff from the provision of affectionate care for less handicapped children. The demands are higher, the skills required are greater and the satisfactions less obvious.

6.   There are many other groups who may need residential care— women with illegitimate babies, adults who, though they are physically or mentally handicapped, can go out to work provided they have the

---

[1] Peter Townsend, *The Last Refuge*, Appendix 6, Table 94A (Routledge & Kegan Paul Ltd., 1962).

support of a secure home background, discharged prisoners facing a new life, or families without the basic skills to make a home for themselves. If we consider these many different groups, it is evident that the staffs of the establishments who look after them have an extremely exacting task. Such work needs special qualities both of mind and of heart—knowledge of the background of the people for whom they are caring, an understanding of the emotional and psychological problems involved and sympathy and tolerance of the human frailties with which they are confronted.

7. But whilst the task is exacting, it is also very rewarding. One of the facts which has emerged forcibly from this enquiry is the amount of happiness and fulfilment experienced by the majority of those engaged in this work. Criticisms of the conditions have been voiced in plenty, and many of these are discussed in following chapters; but it is significant that many of the criticisms have been occasioned by the desire to improve the help given to those in their care, as much as by the desire for an improved status and better remunerated employment.

8. During the course of this enquiry we have talked to a very large number of people—many who attended meetings of the committee in order to give us the benefit of their knowledge and experience, and many whom we have visited in their own establishments in different parts of the country. We have been constantly struck by the amount of sheer goodness we have encountered—by the sympathy and humanity shown by so many in the approach to their jobs, despite difficult conditions, and by readiness to sacrifice their own leisure and interests. Naturally enough, there have been times when we have not fully endorsed the methods employed—for views on such matters vary a good deal—but of two things we all became convinced. First, that the large majority give themselves to their work not only with devotion, but with respect for their fellow human beings who need their help; and second, that the happiness and satisfactions they experience in their work, despite its restrictions and frustrations, stem from their belief that they are doing a job that is so obviously worth while.

9. Certainly nobody ever complained of monotony! Every day brings its problems and its challenge. It is not an easy task to create a harmonious group out of people with diverse backgrounds and diverse temperaments, even when they are young and healthy. To do so when the majority are suffering from disabilities and deprivation is so much the more difficult. But, unlike so much of the work in the modern world, this calls forth all one's capacity and those who undertake it have the additional satisfaction that they can see with their own eyes

B

the results of their efforts in the increased content and happiness of those for whom they work.

10.   We have talked to so many people in this work in the years taken by our enquiry, that it would be foolish to say that we have never heard any single individual express the view that the difficulties are too great to be borne; but there is no doubt that the general impression left with us after these many discussions is that the knowledge that this is a valuable and constructive job is a really important compensation for many of the attendant restrictions and difficulties.

11.   Unfortunately there has not been in the community as a whole a general recognition of the importance of the work nor of the knowledge and skill required to do it well. Too many people have assumed that this is the kind of work that can be done by any reasonably kindly person; the capacity to run a house—see that rooms are kept clean and meals provided—has seemed to be all that is necessary. How wrong is this common conception will become clear when we discuss the nature of the job in the next chapter. But it is largely owing to this widespread fallacy that so little thought has been given to the right training for this work and the conditions of employment that are suitable for it. For, although the competence, skill and knowledge of those undertaking these jobs affects the comfort and happiness of thousands of men, women and children, there is, at present no requirement that training should be taken for it. Courses of training for the staffs of children's Homes have been provided by some voluntary organizations and since 1947 by the Central Training Council in Child Care (Home Office) and these are recognized by an addition to salary. There are also short courses offered by the National Old People's Welfare Council for those taking up work in old people's Homes, but little encouragement is given to people to take this training by offering inducements in the form of salary, status or prospects. As will be seen later, only a small proportion of those now engaged in the work have taken the training offered.

12.   During recent years it has become increasingly clear that the numbers of people able and willing to do this work has not kept pace with demand. The general trend in social policy has been towards the replacement of the large institution by a larger number of smaller establishments in which a more homelike atmosphere can be created. In a later chapter we shall be discussing the problems involved in this trend; at the moment it is only necessary to call attention to the fact that it inevitably has considerable repercussions on staffing. An institution housing some hundreds of people can employ a specialized staff with carefully defined duties and a well-arranged rota of work;

but these cannot easily be introduced in a Home catering for ten or twenty people.

13. At the same time as the demand has increased, there has been a notable growth in alternative employments which demand many of the same qualities as residential work, and this is particularly true in the field of women's employment. Many of these occupations have realized the importance of recognized courses of training in attracting the more able recruits, equipping them with greater competence and also in giving the work both status and prospects; and this has inevitably diminished the reservoir of suitable people available for the running of residential Homes. For whilst residential care work is by no means confined to women, there is no doubt that it offers very many more openings to them than to men. In a later chapter we shall be showing how serious is this dependence on women in a world in which the unmarried woman is rapidly becoming a rarity.

14. The shortage of staff tends to have a cumulative effect. When there are too few people engaged to allow of reasonable times off or anything but snatched holidays, even the kindest and most willing people come to the end of their capacity for overwork and feel forced to give up. And, naturally enough, the longer the hours of work and the more onerous the conditions, the fewer new recruits are ready to come into this field.

15. The problem facing Homes is therefore twofold: it is to attract a sufficient number of the right kind of person in the first place and then to induce them to stay long enough to provide those in their care with a stable environment. This is the problem we decided to investigate; to see if we could find out the main causes of the present situation and whether we could make any proposals that might lead to improvement.

16. After careful consideration we agreed to limit our enquiry to those institutions whose principal purpose is the provision of a home or social education for the many different groups in the community for whom this is required. This is not intended to underestimate the many other functions carried out by the various establishments that we accepted as within our scope; but it does mean that we excluded hospitals and prisons. Indeed some types of accommodation where the categories of resident are clearly within our terms of reference have also received little attention. This ommission was not because we believed that these groups were not important groups, but because in an enquiry of this kind, ranging over so wide and varied a field, it has proved impracticable to examine every group in detail. Moreover we became convinced, as we studied a large number of different kinds of

Home and institution, that our findings and our recommendations have a general application.

17.   Residential accommodation for homeless families provides an example of a significant category to which we have been unable to give detailed study. The ways in which evicted or homeless families are dealt with has attracted a good deal of public attention and concern. The problems presented are often complex and long-term, and efforts at care and rehabilitation vary greatly in method and objectives. On a national basis therefore it appeared impossible to identify any general policy or requirements in terms of staffing. We came to the conclusion that our general proposals about recruitment, conditions of work and especially training apply here also. In practice, any members of staff who work with homeless families, or students who wish to prepare themselves for work with such a group, would be greatly helped by the general training we recommend. They would have the opportunity to take subjects of special relevance and, we anticipate, part of their practical work would be planned with agencies able to provide appropriate experience, such as the Family Service Units.

18.   The main groups we decided to cover are:—

(i) old people; (ii) children and adolescents temporarily or permanently without a normal home (i.e. working boys and girls, mentally and physically handicapped children, including those in residential special schools, delinquent children, including those in approved schools, remand homes and probation hostels); (iii) physically or mentally handicapped adults; (iv) mothers and young children in need of residential accommodation.

19.   Our first need was to find out the facts. There are legal requirements for the registration of most Homes, apart from those run by local authorities. So far as old people's Homes are concerned, there are those provided by voluntary organizations which are non-profit making, and there are those which are run for profit. Both of these must be registered with the local authority, but this does not mean that there is a complete list of them. There are serious problems of definition. A guest house or boarding house or hotel, whose primary purpose in practice is to cater for the elderly, may claim that it does not confine itself to elderly clients, or it may insist that it is prepared to accommodate persons who want 'bed and breakfast' for a night or two, or it may argue that it is none of its business to ask for the birth certificates of those who come to live there. There are, therefore, quite certainly many homes which are principally housing old people but whose liability to register is doubtful or ignored. How many of these there are is unknown, and as matters are at present, there is no way of getting

in touch with them in order to find out. Again, some old people whose circumstances are very similar to those in old people's Homes are in establishments which are registered as nursing homes.

20. Information about children's Homes is almost certainly much more comprehensive. Application to register must be made to the Home Secretary or the Secretary of State for Scotland by any person carrying on, or intending to carry on, a voluntary Home which is not a school within the meaning of the Education Act 1944 or the Education (Scotland) Act 1962. A voluntary Home is defined as one supported wholly or partly by voluntary contributions or endowments and the definition covers 'homes and hostels taking poor children or young persons, other than state or local government institutions maintained out of public funds'. Homes run for profit are not subject to registration, but the person in charge has a duty to notify the local authority of all children admitted for longer than a month.

21. Homes for the mentally disordered and physically handicapped have also to be registered, but as in the case of old people, there are problems of definition between Homes, nursing homes and guest houses.

22. We cannot pretend, therefore, to have compiled completely comprehensive statistics for all the Homes operating in our defined field; but we certainly have knowledge of the great majority of them. We were not, however, primarily concerned to establish the numbers of Homes serving different groups, though this knowledge would be of value. Our primary concern was to discover the way in which the Homes are organized and staffed. How many members of staff are there to care for people in the different groups and in Homes of different sizes? What qualifications or training do they have? Are they married or single? Resident or non-resident? Part-time or full-time? What hours do they work? And how often do they get free time and leave of absence? Is the accommodation agreeable and sufficient? What are the relations between the staff and the residents? Is there an adequate supporting domestic staff? How much are the staff able to mix with the community in the neighbourhood? What is the staff turnover? Who leaves? And who stays? And why? What are the characteristics of the job that are liked? Or disliked? These and similar questions were the ones to which we tried to find answers.

23. When we began, no information was available to enable answers to be given to any of them. Just over ten years ago, Miss S. Clement Brown undertook a survey to review what had happened to students who had been admitted to training in the early years of the establishment, by the Central Training Council in Child Care, of courses started

in 1947 designed for residential staff.[1] This, by definition, was confined to a very small group of persons in one particular field. Then from November 1961 to January 1962 the government Social Survey, at the request of the Home Office, investigated the staffing of residential Homes for children.[2] This was intended to identify some of the reasons for wastage amongst full-time housemothers and assistant house-mothers employed in Local Authority Children's Homes. This information was very valuable, but it only covered some of the staff, and it was confined to Local Authority Homes. Apart from this, little was known.

24. We decided therefore to mount a census of Homes designed to discover as much as we could on these matters. We had many problems to overcome. First and foremost was one of definition. As we were concerned to learn about the 'caring' staff—not the domestic or other grades of employees who might be part of the establishment—we had to try to formulate our questions in such a way as to make clear to respondents the nature of the enquiry. But it is by no means easy to draw a hard and fast line when so often, particularly in very small children's Homes, the caring staff also do a good deal of domestic work, and the person in charge may be responsible for most, if not all, of the cooking: or in some approved schools and residential special schools, where teachers undertake some of the caring and home-making functions.

25. Our second problem stemmed from the great variety in the organisation and control of the Homes and the consequent difficulty of phrasing questions in such a way that people could answer them clearly and directly. These and other problems are explained in Chapter IV which gives details of how the census was carried out and tabulates some of the results.

26. It will be seen that we cannot claim that we have compiled a complete and comprehensive and absolutely accurate survey of the whole field. What we *can* claim, however, is that for the first time it is possible to get a general picture of the residential care field and a conspectus of some of the problems involved in staffing it. Indeed, despite the legal requirements of registration which enabled much to be known of the numbers of Homes in existence, there has never before been any attempt to add together the numbers providing for different groups of those in need: and it is probable that even those who have given much care and thought to particular groups will be astonished

[1] S. Clement Brown, 'The Training of Houseparents for work in Children's Homes'. Dec. 1956. Nuffield College Library, Oxford (unpublished).
[2] *Staffing of Local Authority Residential Homes for Children 1961–1962*, Government Social Survey. Published by H.M.S.O.

to find how large is the total number when all sectors are taken into account. In the whole of our field we know of over 7,000 Homes, caring for close on a quarter of a million people.

27. The size and character became the essential framework of our enquiry; but we needed more than this. It is idle to imagine that one can get real insight into any human problem by figures alone; and we decided to visit as many Homes as we could, in different localities and providing for various groups of people. We wanted to see for ourselves the conditions provided and to talk to the men and women who were doing the work and try to see the situation through their eyes. For this reason, we arranged for small groups of committee members—four or five at a time—to spend a few days in a centre and visit as wide a range of the institutions in the neighbourhood as was possible in the time. To extend the scope, we divided ourselves into twos and threes, and went on different rounds and we reassembled in the evenings to exchange our knowledge and impressions and discuss the ideas that had occurred to us during our visits.

28. We are glad to have this opportunity of expressing our gratitude to all who helped us during these visits. Local authorities and voluntary organizations did all in their power to arrange the programmes that we outlined to them, and in the Homes we were always received with the greatest kindness and goodwill. We had feared that there might be occasions on which the assistant staff might feel some diffidence in voicing their problems and criticisms in the presence of those in charge of the Home and we asked for opportunities—for example, over a cup of tea or coffee—to talk to them without constraint. This opportunity was invariably granted and we all felt that we had gained knowledge and insight by these conversations.

29. At the outset of our enquiry we issued a statement to the press giving the scope of our work and inviting organizations and individuals to send us written memoranda or suggest themselves as oral witnesses. In addition we wrote to a very large number of people—both those who could speak for organizations or statutory authorities and those who might have valuable experience which they would be willing to share with us—inviting them to attend one of our meetings to discuss the problems with us. We received a very large body of evidence in this way and arranged 36 sessions at which individuals or representatives of organizations came to discuss these matters with us. The list of those who helped in this way is to be found in Appendix A. In all we have held 45 main Committee meetings, most of them lasting a full day and several times a whole weekend, in order to discuss the various points of view and attempt to reach a consensus of opinion.

30.   As we progressed in our discussion we became unanimous in the strength of our conviction that the problem would never be solved unless comprehensive training for residential work could be established.

31.   The work itself calls on so much knowledge and skill that it cannot be expected that people should be able to undertake it successfully without adequate preparation. But it is also important that the lack of a recognized credential tends to lower its status in competition with similar kinds of work for which there are established courses of training. We set up, therefore, the Training Sub-Committee under Dr Gibbs' chairmanship to which reference has already been made in the Foreword. Their proposals were brought constantly before the full committee for detailed discussion and amendment and there is general agreement that the substance of the chapter which embodies the results of these discussions is one of the most important parts of this Report.

32.   Certain matters have so persistently threaded all our discussions that some reference must be made to them here. There are three that stand out with special prominence.

33.   The first relates to the general attitude to residential care of a large part of the community. With the exception of those whose own work brings them into close contact with residential Homes there is little understanding of the nature of the job or of the skill and responsibility involved. It may be that the trend towards smaller Homes has contributed somewhat to this lack of appreciation. When one is confronted by a very large building, housing hundreds of people and with an appropriately large staff, it is not difficult to realize that those in charge have a big job to do. Even though people may not have sufficient insight to appreciate that, even here, the most important part of the task is in the field of human relationships, it is obvious that the administration and organization need special capacity. But to many people, control of a small Home seems more or less the same sort of job as that done by any housewife with a fairly large family and little is understood of the special skill and knowledge demanded by it.

34.   The nagging belief that the qualities needed in this responsible and important work are grossly under-estimated by the majority of the community is a constant source of discontent and frustration to those who devote themselves to it. This was one of the recurring themes, both of the written memoranda submitted to us and of the oral evidence we received. Indeed, it is possible that the almost universal demand for the provision of suitable courses of training made by practically everybody who wrote or spoke to us drew part of its strength from the anxiety to gain general recognition that something more is needed than

the motherly woman or the economical housekeeper—valuable as these qualities are in any residential worker.

35. In a later chapter we have gone into some detail in our analysis of the nature of the job because we want to make clear that the task of making a Home for such groups as we have earlier referred to calls for knowledge, understanding and a variety of skills which cannot be assumed to exist, without training, in everybody who happens to be willing to undertake the work. Here is a profession which, in common with all other professions, demands both certain individual aptitudes and a body of disciplined knowledge and developed skills which can be acquired only by formal courses of preparation.

But is it, in fact, *one* profession? Or could it become so? This is the second matter that constantly exercised our minds. We found in practice that most people concerned with residential care devote themselves to one, and only one, section of the field. Some look after children, some after mother and baby Homes, others after the old or the handicapped. It is rare to find people who move from one kind of Home to another. Is this inevitable? Are people always so specialized in their sympathy and concern? Or is this high degree of specialization one consequence of the present way in which Homes are provided and controlled? And even if some would always choose to keep within one kind of work, are not the knowledge and skill required by them more or less the same?

37. The question is important. If the answer to it is that there is one all-embracing profession—'residential care'—two consequences result. First, it is possible to provide courses of training which offer a common basis for all engaged in it, whatever further specialized knowledge or experience they may need for their particular field of interest; and second, movement from one section to another offers very much wider opportunities for those whose increasing knowledge and experience lead them to seek posts with greater responsibility than can be available in any one part of the whole field.

39. The third general topic which has influenced our thinking on almost all aspects of the subject is the effect on staffing of the recent trend towards smaller Homes. 'Large' and 'small' are relative terms. There is a world of difference between the old type of barracks institution with a thousand old people living in it and the pleasant 'villa' with thirty or so; but there are many points in-between. And what is small for one group of people is large for another. For example, the need of young children for a warm, cosy environment and an individual adult with whom they can establish a secure relationship demands a smaller Home than that of handicapped adults who seek

maximum independence and who may enjoy the greater variety of companionship afforded by one that is rather larger. Even in our social policy, 'small' and 'large' are constantly given different connotations as we learn more of the psycholgical and emotional problems involved in living in a group.

40.   Wherever we put the dividing line, the staffing needs inevitably vary from one size to another; and it is, unfortunately, impossible to take it for granted that the size of Home which might provide the happiest environment for the people in care, is necessarily the same as that which would allow the hours and conditions of employment which would enable the staff to live full, happy and rounded lives. If we wished to be realistic, therefore, we had constantly to keep in mind the need to reconcile conflicting interests.

41.   All these problems are discussed in greater detail in later chapters. They are mentioned here because they conditioned so much of our thinking and affected so many of our recommendations.

42.   One of our particular problems, rather different in character from those mentioned above has been that of terminology. We have tried, as far as possible, to avoid the word 'institution' but we are aware that 'Home' does not accurately cover the schools which we have included in our survey. Similarly we have not found it easy to settle on any acceptable word for those who are being cared for. 'Inmate' was disliked by us but it was difficult to find any more attractive word that was sufficiently comprehensive. We therefore agreed to use the word 'resident' although we recognize that this has a certain ambiguity because it might be thought to include those members of the staff who live in the Home. However, when we use the word resident in this Report, unless the context obviously indicates a different meaning, we refer to the people in care. Again, there has been the problem of a name by which to refer to the person in charge of a Home, or to his deputy and assistants, which does not carry the wrong associations. 'Matron', the most usual, is too closely associated with the nursing profession and we are anxious to dissociate the work and qualities of the word, admirable as those are, from those of the 'Home-maker'. 'Warden' though an honourable title in university circles has an unfortunate connotation in the general mind and 'Superintendent' has too formal and authoritarian a sound. So we have been compelled to use the somewhat clumsy terms 'those in charge' or 'Heads of Homes'.

2

THE NATURE OF THE JOB

1. We have emphasised the skill and knowledge required in this work. Why are these so essential? What is the nature of the work to be done?

2. In the first chapter stress was laid on the fact that the people in residential care are by no means a cross-section of the population as a whole. They are those for whom the expanding domiciliary services are not adequate because of characteristics or circumstances which make it difficult for them to live independently or to be cared for in an ordinary family. As the figures in our Census show, the old people in residential homes are generally far beyond the normal age of retirement (65 for a man and 60 for a woman). In fact, just about half are over 80 years of age and many of them have some degree of infirmity or are slightly confused. And it is just at this difficult stage in their lives that they are asked to adjust to a completely different pattern of existence.

3. One basic fact has to be kept in mind—that even the best residential Home is likely to be ranked as second best in the mind of those who come into it. It cannot replace the independence a person enjoys in his own home or give what an affectionate family can provide. Everything is different from what he has been accustomed to for so long. The rooms may be warm and bright and prettily decorated, the chairs comfortable, the food good and plentiful. But they are different and take getting used to. And one's new companions are not those whom one has known all one's life, who understand the names that crop up in the conversation or recognize the references to past experiences. It is a sad thing not only to suffer the infirmities of old age but to find oneself amongst strangers at a time of life when it is difficult to make new friends.

4. But even if an old person finds it impossible to continue to live in the normal community, there is no need to assume that he immediately becomes completely incapable of all independent action. He still has his own individuality and wants to preserve his privacy and his own place in the world. In his life prior to his entering the home he has been accustomed to making his own decisions and acting on them, and,

provided he does not infringe the freedom of others, there is no reason why he should not continue to do so. Despite physical infirmity he may still be capable of managing his own affairs, of choosing his own interests and selecting his own friends.

5.   Difficult behaviour and childishness are ways in which some people express their unhappiness and it depends very greatly on the staff how soon old people adjust themselves to their circumstances and evolve a new pattern of living. Those who look after the elderly have to try to steer a course between over-protection on the one hand and lack of needed care and support on the other; to urge some to attempt independent action when they may be too ready to give up, and help others to adjust to an acceptance of dependance. And what makes all this the more difficult, is that these people, each faced with his individual problem, are all living in a community.

6.   The chief work of those in charge of a Home is to create a harmonious group out of men and women brought together by nothing more than the hazards of circumstances, and to do it in such a way that whilst each feels secure in the care given him, he is yet free to live as full and as independent a life as is allowed by his physical or mental limitations. At the same time care must be taken not to isolate the Home from the neighbourhood. Much of the pleasure of life of those who can no longer be very active comes from the sense of still being in touch with all that is going on; of friendly gossip with neighbours and relatives and the stimulus that is given by seeing different faces. It is only if the staff are pleasantly welcoming to visitors that those who live in the locality are likely to be willing to provide this stimulus for those who are too infirm to venture out themselves. To do this requires a good deal of knowledge of the human mind and emotions as well as a tolerant sympathy with other people's difficulties.

7.   However hard it may be to do this when one is concerned with a group of elderly people, it is even more so when those in one's charge are children. Here it is not enough to give the child or adolescent a sense of security by the extension of simple friendship or to try to heal the hurts suffered in separation from his home, but it is necessary to help him to develop his own personality and capacity in whatever direction they may lead. A sheltered and comfortable home is not enough, for eventually all children must learn to live in the world and stand on their own feet. They have to be helped to take their share in ordinary activities, to learn from their mistakes, to adapt to the rough and tumble of schools and the various leisure time occupations. In these days of heightened consciousness of the value of individual personality and of the changing relationship of the generations to one

another, it is difficult enough to be a good parent to one's own children. To provide for a whole group of children something that does not pretend to be a parent-child relationship, but yet gives them a similar sense of warmth and security and 'belonging' is all the more difficult. Yet this is what the staff of a children's Home must try to do. And this means more than ensuring that the children are cheerful and healthy and are ready to take a part in the life of the Home; it involves the willingness to recognize that, for some children, breaking the rules and even a certain amount of 'cussedness' are an essential element in the strenuous process of 'growing up'; and sadness and depression call for great understanding.

8.   Mrs Clare Winnicott expressed this particularly well when she wrote: 'Children need from the residential worker something direct and real, and treatment surely lies in the worker's ability to provide for them real experiences of good care, comfort and control. This good care will include timing that can allow personal experiences to be completed and a sense of achievement attained. It will include recognizing that each child has individual needs, and attempting to meet the needs of each if only in a token way. The token can be used because behind it is both the recognition of the need and the will to meet it. These good experiences are not only the stuff of life, but the stuff "that dreams are made on," and have the power to become part of the child's inner psychic reality, correcting the past and creating the future.'[1]

9.   To create ties with the locality is a good deal easier as far as children are concerned than for the elderly; for those of school age attend the normal schools and have a chance of making friends outside the Home. But here there is the much more difficult task of gaining the cooperation of the parents and sharing the children's affections with them. Parents can be hostile and critical and the staff often find it hard to accept adverse comments from those they believe to have been careless or neglectful of their children. Most children love their own parents, however inadequate they may have proved, and it is no easy matter for those who are giving them devoted care to recognize and encourage this natural feeling.

10.   Much of what has been said about the work of those looking after the aged and the young applies equally to those who have the adult handicapped in their care. But here again there are problems peculiar to them. The difficulty of drawing a line of demarcation between overprotection and neglect of special needed care is here particularly pronounced. For those who are handicapped there is not only the need to learn a skill that may open the doors of employment to them but those

---

[1] Clare Winnicott, *Child Care and Social Work* (Codicote Press, 1964).

who care for them have the much more delicate task of providing the constant encouragement and support that gradually builds up their confidence in their own capacity to venture into the outside world.

11. There are some people who have asked why one should make so much more of the qualities needed for this kind of work than those shown by so many families both for their older members and their young children. After all, it is argued, most of us have to face both these demands at different times during our lives—to provide a pleasant and helpful environment for the elderly and a secure, but not inhibiting, home for the young, and there are many families with a handicapped member. Why then, should one consider the work of those in residential institutions as something out of the ordinary, needing both more knowledge and skill? And why should we feel such concern for their conditions of employment and living accommodation? This misconception, that residential care is just the same as the work of every family, but on a larger scale, is so common that it is worth considering in some detail.

12. First, there is the time element to take into account. A family may have two or even four, elderly members in need of special care; but in the nature of things there is a limit to the number of years that this places a responsibility on the younger members. In an old people's Home, on the other hand, one difficult situation follows another in an unending sequence. When one member of the group reaches the end of his life, another at once takes his place and calls for the same care and thought from those who look after him.

Similarly in a children's Home there is the problem of the amount and the continuity of the care needed. It would be a very exceptional family in which all the young people were emotionally disturbed or handicapped in some way. The special attention demanded by one is, in a sense, compensated for by the other 'normal' members of the family. And even if the family is much larger than is usual nowadays, the period of complete dependence finally comes to an end. But in a children's Home a very large proportion are disturbed in some degree, if only by the break in family life, and the period of dependence never comes to an end.

13. Most parents accept the fact that they must be 'on duty' for twenty-four hours of the day when their children are very young and for this time they are generally willing to subordinate everything to the needs of the child—their own interests, their leisure time activities, seeing their friends and so on. They know that this period of sacrifice lasts only a few years and changes as the children reach adolescence and greater independence. But those in charge of a children's Home have no

such time of freedom to look forward to. For them it remains always the early days of childhood and it is not reasonable to expect that the complete subordination of one's own life which may be gladly undertaken for two or three years, can continue for twenty or thirty on the same basis.

14. So far we have spoken only of the qualities needed to provide happily for those for whose benefit the Home exists, but it must be remembered that the staff must also be considered, and it is often much easier to recognize the claims of those for whom one is caring than those of one's fellow-workers. There are many occasions when the situation itself throws up special problems. For example, when the Home is small there may be a married couple in charge and only one other member of staff. Unless special care is taken to accept her in the family circle—and this in itself detracts from the sense of carefree leisure of the husband and wife—she may feel excluded and lonely. But even when the staff is large enough to enable friendships to be formed, there are many difficult problems. We are now beginning, very slowly, to appreciate the major part played in industrial and commercial enterprises by the constant interaction of human personality and, indeed, one of the most important elements in the training of managers in industry is now recognized to be in this field. How much more important it is, then, when the nature of the work is such as to make exceptional calls on sympathy, understanding and tolerance.

15. This is not a problem simply of a closed community of people forced to spend both working and leisure time in each other's company; for, as will be shown in a later chapter, a large proportion of the staff are not themselves resident and this proportion is likely to grow in the future. It is inherent in the situation and is aggravated by the circumstances in which it must be carried on. Some of the difficulties are obvious because they are shared by any occupation which demands shift working. Those living in the Home must be cared for at all times and this means that members of staff must be prepared to give up some of their evenings and weekends when they would like to be with their families and friends or pursuing their own interests. But other difficulties are not so apparent. For example, when a married couple have their own young children, it is hard for them to judge how much time they should devote to them without taking away time and thought from the children in the Home. Parents cannot be expected to divest themselves of their normal parental feelings, nor would it be right for them to do so; but it is not easy to tread the narrow path between making too great a distinction between their own children and the others, or too little. And it is fairly certain that whatever they do, there

will be other members of the staff, looking at them with watchful, and, perhaps, critical eyes. This does not make for simple and easy staff relationships.

16.   Mention was made in the last chapter of the Survey made for the Home Office into the staffing of residential Homes for children. It is interesting and significant that the investigation into the reasons for which people left their posts, showed that a quarter of those who left for 'Reasons Related to the Job' (i.e. not on account of retirement or marriage or domestic circumstances) gave 'friction and incompatibility with other members of staff' as their reasons. Our own Census does not allow us to draw any valid conclusions in this matter for, unlike the Home Office Survey which was able to get its information through personal interviews, we had to rely on written answers to a questionnaire and most respondents are usually a little more unwilling to commit their views to paper. But just about a third, both of those leaving old people's Homes and those leaving children's Homes, gave 'leaving the profession' as the explanation of quitting the job and though it is not possible to guess how many of those left the field on account of their experience of working with uncongenial colleagues, it is, at least, likely that this played some part. There is certainly no doubt that the creation and maintenance of happy relationships amongst the staff is an important and essential part of the work of those in charge of a Home, both in its own right and because of its indirect influence on the happiness of those for whom the Home exists.

17.   What qualities then, are needed to do well the kind of work we have been describing? If we list those we think important it might seem that we are indulging in fantastic day-dreaming and that only a phalanx of archangels could possibly match up to our requirements. We are well aware of this and say, at once, that we do not expect to find any large number of people who possess all these qualities to the highest degree. But we are convinced that, whilst it may be rash to believe that there are many with *all* these characteristics, there are, fortunately, a very considerable number who have some of them; and we are equally convinced that many of these qualities which may exist only as potentialities can be greatly developed by training and experience.

18.   In one sense, those who undertake this work are more likely than most to have the aptitudes we are looking for. Though it is unhappily true that some are attracted to this work for the wrong reasons, the majority of people who come into this work and who remain in it for more than a very short period, generally have a strong liking for their fellow human beings and have compassion for those suffering from some misfortune or infirmity. And though liking and sympathy are not

enough, they are a good beginning. There are, however, many who choose to work, as the saying is 'with people rather than with things' who yet do not possess the insight and humility and the respect for the individuality of those in their care which would make them refrain from a too authoritarian attitude towards them. The person who feels certain that she knows what is good for others is not likely to create a happy friendly home in which those in residence can live, as far as possible, according to their own preferences. And similarly the 'fuss-pot', however hardworking and competent she may be, is more likely to produce a spotlessly clean and efficient establishment rather than a relaxed, friendly, home-like atmosphere.

19. Energy and resourcefulness, the capacity to cope with the unexpected without flurry and to take decisions when definite action is called for are all important attributes; but serenity and a respect for others are equally outstanding essentials. Yet, although these qualities of temperament are so much needed, they do not, of themselves, give the knowledge of complex human personalities and relationships on which really helpful and constructive care must be founded. The ability to learn and comprehend something of the workings of the mind and the emotions and the ways in which people's behaviour and ideas have been fashioned by their lives, their families and their social background are the necessary corollary to the qualities of character we have demanded. There are marked differences in patterns of behaviour in different regions and social groups and manners which are perfectly normal to one group may strike those who are more familiar with another in quite a different light. Some understanding of the great variety of ways in which people are accustomed to express themselves and to carry on their day-to-day activities leads to tolerance and avoids friction. It is not enough for those in charge to develop this sympathetic approach which is founded on knowledge and understanding, but also all those who come in close daily contact with those being cared for; and much depends on the ability of those in charge to help their colleagues to appreciate the nature of the problems with which they are faced, in creating a happy community.

20. It may be a matter of surprise that no mention has yet been made of what, at first sight, might have been considered the first requisite; i.e. the technical skills of home-making. This is not because we underestimate the importance of these but because they are more obvious and more easily acquired than the subtler ones involved in creating a friendly and happy community. But they are, of course essential. Running a home for a family requires a whole battery of skills if it is to be well done and these are needed even more when there are many

people of different tastes to be served and expenditure must be kept within the limits prescribed by the controlling authority. Careful budgeting, choice of varied and appetizing meals, avoidance of rigid rules, taste in furnishings and the organization of staff duties on a fair and acceptable basis are all needed if the Home is to function in a reasonably care-free way. What makes this work even more difficult is the necessity to get the cooperation of as many as possible of those living in the Home in its running. It is very often much easier to do things for people than to persuade, or to allow them, to take a share. But whatever the groups for whom the Home exists—whether old people, children, the handicapped or others—playing a part in the chores of one's own home is both a satisfaction in itself and also an essential element in the creation amongst a number of people of the feeling that they are living together rather than simply being 'housed' together. The competent housewife may often be irritated by the slow movements of the old or the clumsiness of the handicapped but to encourage them to share in the work is as much a part of the 'home-making' skill as careful budgeting or supervision of the preparation of nourishing meals.

21. Even in a fairly small Home, however, there are other members of staff who care for those living there. There are, indeed, generally two categories to be distinguished. The first comprises the heads and deputy heads and others in charge of groups, of whom we have mainly been speaking in this chapter. The second consists of assistants whose work is to look after those in the Home, and the part-time workers, generally married women living in the locality, who are prepared to care for those in the Home for a part of each week, but whose principal concern is the care of their own households and families. It would be unrealistic to expect them all to possess the range and level of qualities and know-ledge that we have spoken of as necessary for the more responsible posts. Nevertheless it is they who often have the closest and most continuous daily contact with the residents and their way of carrying out their duties can make all the difference between content and misery for those in their care. Whilst one cannot demand that their know-ledge of human relationships should be as wide as that of the senior staff, it is important that they should be taught to add to kindly treat-ment, a genuine respect for the independence and individuality of those for whom they are caring, and to be aware of their social and personal problems.

22. Many of these qualities on which we have laid stress have developed through experience amongst those at present undertaking this work. But this development could take place more rapidly and

thoroughly and many unhappy blunders could be avoided if those with the natural capacities had the advantage of specific training to enable them to do this exacting job.

3

HISTORICAL BACKGROUND

1.   At any period of time, the residential establishment reflects what the community wants for those in need and therefore what kind of care the staff are expected to give them. Changes in social philosophy very directly affect the job the staff are called on to do. The nature of residential care as we have described it in Chapter 2 is of an entirely different order from what was expected of the nineteenth century workhouse master.

2.   Residential communities originated in two sharply differentiated impulses. The first was primarily the need to protect society from the lunatic, the thief or the sturdy vagabond, for in spite of the views held about individual responsibility, the community was not prepared to let them die; so in the seventeenth century poor law legislation set up the first workhouses and poorhouses. The second impulse was the Christian duty of charity to the unfortunate, which had started long before with the hospitals and schools run by monastic orders or founded by lay benevolence, and which has continued and developed ever since, although not by so clear cut a line as the statutory provisions.

3.   During the eighteenth and nineteenth centuries, the mixed general workhouse became almost the only accommodation provided by the state for society's casualties—the young and the old, the infirm and able-bodied, and many of the mentally ill and defective. Fear of encouraging the able-bodied poor to live on the rates led to strict deterrent discipline and the principle of 'less eligibility'; that is, that all inmates regardless of sickness or age must be worse off than the poorest unskilled wage earner. In such circumstances the staff were not expected to give what we would call care to the inmates. Indeed, apart from the workhouse master and his wife there was no staff. The work of the establishment was carried out by paupers, and the sick and aged were tended—or were not—by their fellow inmates. Pauper children were put out to work almost as soon as they could walk in order not to be a burden on the ratepayers. It was only after a series of scandals in the

late nineteenth century that paid nurses were employed to nurse the pauper sick, but even in 1909 the Poor Law Commission drew attention to the work still being done in most workhouses by the pauper assistants, irrespective of their fitness.

4. At the same time, private individuals and religious organizations pioneered new kinds of residential care, especially for children. Men like Barnardo, Stephenson or Sidney Turner in England, or Thomas Guthrie in Scotland; the Anglican, Presbyterian, Roman Catholic and Free Churches, or the Salvation Army, not only set up Homes, but helped to make the public aware of the gaps in the statutory provisions. By modern standards, much of this Victorian charity may have been harsh, but these pioneers and the dedicated staff they gathered round them were trying to do something new. They were trying to turn those they cared for into useful citizens and unlike the workhouses, they were concerned with rehabilitation rather than deterrence.

5. The twentieth century has seen a gradual change in social attitude to the unfortunate. The Poor Law Commission of 1909, and its parallel Commission in Scotland, roused the interest of the community in the plight of its poorer members and so gave rise to a very considerable amount of discussion on the ways they could be helped. The result was a burst of social legislation which laid the foundation for the later welfare state. The 'Children's Charter' of 1908 and the social welfare legislation of the same period, followed during the 1920s and 1930s by a number of government reports on different groups—defective children, the mentally disturbed, the handicapped, young offenders and so on—led to a growth in public concern which was accelerated by the mass unemployment of the thirties. This created problems of poverty and sickness too big for the existing statutory and voluntary organizations. Then the experiences of the Second World War fundamentally changed the attitude of society to 'the poor'. Bombing and evacuation drew attention to the plight of old people no longer able to look after themselves; evacuated children billeted on private families or cared for in small groups revealed a state of deprivation hitherto largely concealed in the slums of industrial cities. 'Evacuation . . . revealed to the whole people the black spots of its social life.'[1] For the first time, too, members of the middle classes found themselves at the receiving end of the state's provisions.

6. These changes naturally had a profound effect on the residential institution and therefore on the job the staff had to do. As a result of the new policy implied in the phrase 'community care,' more people were kept out of residential care, so that those who were in residential

[1] *Economist*, 1st May, 1943, quoted in Professor R. Titmuss, 'Social Policy'.

Homes were likely to be frailer, more disturbed or more delinquent. As we have said in Chapter 1, in the last twenty years residential staff have had a more difficult job to do. Also, the general rise in material standards and the growing understanding of the importance of social and psychological factors has meant that people are no longer satisfied with standards of care which seemed adequate in the 1930s.[1]

7. But the most important factors affecting the residential care of children were the government enquiries into the care of children in 1946.[2] The Reports of these enquiries gave preference to the care of children in private families. This implied that staff needed special ability in order to receive children while individual decisions about their future were made, and it meant that Homes tended to be used for more difficult children, less likely to settle in private families.

8. The Reports also laid great emphasis on the care of children in small groups, and the necessity to have trained staff to look after them. They considered that the most suitable Home for children was the small family group, preferably in charge of a married couple, whether it was a 'cottage' or 'flat' within a large establishment, or an independent household similar to those of the neighbours. The Committees were influenced by the comparative intimacy and naturalness of the family group Home, where the wife was in charge whilst the husband probably followed his own occupation. Here the children would be more closely in touch with the experiences of everyday life. Similarly, they recommended that young children in nurseries should be cared for in small groups.

9. The Curtis Committee was so concerned that there should be adequate preparation for those undertaking responsibility for children that they published their recommendations about training in advance of their main report. The voluntary organizations had given evidence of the value of training because they had run training courses for some time, in one case extending over a period of nearly fifty years.[3] (For the Approved Schools training had already been agreed by the Reynold's Committee[4] and was later urged by the Underwood Committee,[5] for the staff concerned with handicapped children.) As a result

[1] e.g. Janet Hitchman, *King of the Barbareens*, for a description of institutional care of children in the 1930's.

[2] The Curtis Committee in England (*Report of the Care of Children Committee*, September 1946, Cmnd 6922.) and the Clyde Committee in Scotland (*Report on Homeless Children*, 1946, Cmnd 6911).

[3] Wilson, Audrey, *Progress in Child Care*, National Children's Home, Highbury Park, London, N.5. The Convocation Lecture, 1957.

[4] Home Office: Reynolds, B. J., *Conditions of Service and Qualifications of Approved Schools Staff*, 1946 (Out of Print).

[5] Ministry of Education: *Report of the Committee on Maladjusted Children*, pp. 126-131. H.M.S.O. 1955.

of the Curtis and Clyde Committees' recommendations, training courses lasting fourteen months were set up by the Central Training Council and similar courses were set up in Scotland. The Committees' views were incorporated in the Children Act, 1948 both in England and in Scotland. This led to a very great increase in the number of children boarded out with foster parents in England and Wales—from 35 per cent of those in Local Authority care in 1949 to 52 per cent in 1965,[1] and in both countries to a drive to provide new residential Homes, most of them small. Nowadays over 70 per cent of Local Authority children's Homes are small family group Homes for five to twelve children. The responsibilities, the social life, and in some respects the status of houseparents in charge of such small Homes is very different from the head of the large children's Home, and they are providing a different kind of relationship with the children in their care.

10. In the twenty years since the publication of these Reports, doubts have grown as to whether the small family group Home is always the best for all children and provides the best framework in which all staff can work. Some people now consider that the most important thing is to have a great variety of kinds of provision, to cater for the needs of different children and the different qualities and preferences of staff.

11. In 1963 the Children and Young Persons Act empowered local authorities to employ their resources to keep families together wherever possible so that children should not be taken into care unnecessarily. This is likely to have a significant effect on the nature of the work of residential Homes. They are increasingly used for the care of children for undetermined, but in some cases quite short, periods to relieve family strain. Some of these children come into care because of serious behaviour problems in their homes. In all cases, the parents as well as children need help and guidance which must be given by residential workers working in partnership with child care officers.

12. For old people's Homes, too, policy since 1948 has moved towards the provision of small Homes of about 50 residents. The Ministry of Health's annual report of 1948-9 said that local authorities were busy planning and opening small comfortable old people's Homes 'where the old master and inmate relationship is being replaced by one more nearly approaching a hotel manager and his guests.' This was an over-optimistic statement. Pressure on accommodation has been such that not all of the old public assistance institutions have yet been closed, although they have been much improved. 27,000 people were still in

---

[1] In Scotland, where the tradition of fostering was already more firmly established, the corresponding figures remained steady at about 60 per cent.

1965 resident in them (although this was only about half as many as in 1949). It was also over-optimistic in that it under-estimated the number of very frail who are in residential care today and who need much more skilled care from the staff than a hotel manager provides. Nevertheless, there is today a real and increasingly successful attempt to create small and comfortable Homes. Over 60 per cent of those in local authority care in 1965 were in Homes with under 70 places.

13. Homes for the socially inadequate, the sub-normal and the mentally ill have been started only in the last few years, and are still in an experimental stage. They are on the whole small as they have arisen in the period when small Homes are generally accepted as desirable.

14. In spite of difficulties in the way of providing the best kind of care, what we have today is a new attitude—a recognition of the need to do things for individuals rather than categories of people. The whole social provision depends on classifying the common elements in a situation as a basis for social legislation, but having done this the real dilemma is somehow to care for people as individuals while recognizing the category into which they fall. It is these changes in social philosophy which are characteristic of our thinking today compared with the past; and these changes very directly affect the job the staff have to do because we are trying to achieve something altogether more subtle and more worth-while than merely providing a roof over people's heads and adequate food and warmth.

4

THE SURVEY ENQUIRY

1. We wanted to find out as much as possible about the staff employed in residential establishments and so we conducted our 'census'. The Census Sub-Committee set up under the chairmanship of Dr Mark Adams to do this, immediately came up against a number of problems.

2. First, the many different types of Homes to be covered made it difficult to draw up a single form suitable for all of them—for example, the age range of residents in a school is very different from those in old people's Homes. We therefore used three forms of questionnaire, one for old people's Homes, one for schools and one for children's Homes and other Homes. The questions on each were identical, but the spaces for replies were divided differently. Second, our enquiry was concerned only with the caring staff and with others only insofar as their work was devoted to residents. Where, as is so often the case, staff had mixed duties, we had to give instructions regarding definitions. In Part I of the questionnaire we asked for information about all staff. In Part II we asked about caring staff only. Third, there were the Homes which are run under some form of religious discipline, for example, the Catholic and Anglican Orders or the Salvation Army. They do not have the same kind of staffing problems as the main body of residential establishments and therefore, unless they employed considerable numbers of lay caring staff, we excluded them from our enquiry. This means that the response rate for old people's Homes and children's Homes run by voluntary organizations appears to be low, because although we could exclude these Homes from our 'census', we were unable to know their numbers with sufficient accuracy to exclude them from the total number of voluntary Homes.

3. We decided to conduct a small pilot survey to test the questionnaires, and as a result we found a number of difficulties and ambiguities. We therefore reconstructed the questionnaire, and tested it with a second larger pilot survey and modified it again as a result. The final questionnaire is shown in Appendix B. We cannot claim we were able

to overcome all the problems. The complexity of the field of enquiry would make it impossible in the time at our disposal. But two pilot surveys enabled us to phrase our questions in a form which the majority of respondents understood.

4. Our next problem was concerned with distribution. Our enquiry covered the whole of the U.K.—England, Wales, Scotland and Northern Ireland—and the administrative bodies in these various countries are not identical. We were extremely fortunate to gain the co-operation of the local authorities and the voluntary organizations responsible for running residential Homes, each of whom undertook to distribute our questionnaires to all the Homes under their respective controls.

5. There is, however, a considerable number of residential institutions which do not come under the control of these organizations. Where central lists existed, for example, for approved schools, mother and baby homes and so on, we sent the questionnaire direct to the head of the institution. In addition, local authorities were asked either to send out questionnaires on our behalf to the private and voluntary homes in their areas, which were not covered by the large voluntary organizations, or to give us a list of their names and addresses. But as we have explained already in Chapter 1, there are problems of definition. For example, some Homes returned the questionnaires but explained that all caring staff were nurses and therefore were not within our scope. Second, there was some double counting—two local authorities which used a voluntary Home both sent forms to it, or some voluntary Homes got forms direct from us or their own headquarters, and from the local authorities. Few filled in the questionnaires twice, but this accounts for the fact that we sent out more questionnaires than there are Homes and schools.

6. Considering the difficulties of this enquiry, the return rate was extraordinarily high. In some categories we got almost a 100 per cent return, and in most we got between 60 per cent and 70 per cent. In all, we had 4,343 usable questionnaires returned, which means that our survey covers a high proportion of the whole field—probably about 60 per cent. This represents information about more staff in residential accommodation than has ever before been collected together.

7. The only real gap is that which concerns old people's Homes run for profit (i.e. the category we call 'private' in the survey). Here the response rate was only about 10 per cent. Many of these Homes did not return our questionnaires, but sometimes some local authorities did not send out our quesionnaires to private Homes registered with them and did not furnish us with their names and addresses. We therefore had no means of sending questionnaires to them.

8. The questions we asked can be seen in Appendix B; the information refers to residents and to staff on the pay roll on November 30, 1963.

9. We are not publishing in this Report all the detailed information we gained from this enquiry. To do so would increase by a very great amount the cost of publication which would not be justified by the nature of the information available. The full tables we had tabulated are available in the National Council of Social Service and a further copy is in the National Institute for Social Work Training. Those especially interested can have access to them there, or a duplicated copy of the tables can be purchased from the National Council of Social Service.[1]

10. The answers to certain questions have not been tabulated at all. This is true, for example, for the age of the building (Question 4). We had anticipated that there might be a significant difference between the rate of turnover, the satisfaction or dissatisfaction with accommodation and so on between staff working in old buildings and those working in modern ones, but our preliminary sifting of the information showed there were few significant correlations. There was other information not tabulated—e.g. information about establishments catering for homeless families—because the total replies received were too small to classify.

11. The material that has been coded has been analysed and tabulated in four broad groups. The two biggest groups are old people's Homes and children's Homes. These we have analysed by size, dividing them into 5 size groups and by type—local authority Homes and voluntary Homes, and in the case of old people, private Homes as well.

12. The third group are approved schools, remand Homes and Special Schools and the fourth is the rest—nurseries for under-fives, reception Homes, hostels for adolescents, mother and baby Homes, Homes for physically handicapped adults and Homes for mentally handicapped adults. These two groups we have analysed according to each type of school or Home, but the numbers were too small for them to be further sub-divided by size or between local authority Homes and voluntary Homes.

13. The results of these analyses will be found on the following pages. In all cases, the figures apply to the U.K.

I. SURVEY OF OLD PEOPLE'S HOMES

14. About half of all old people's Homes in the U.K. are run by local authorities, and two-thirds of the old people in residential care are in

[1] A full list of the tables available for consultation is given in Appendix B.

these local authority Homes. In our survey the response rate from these Homes was very much greater than from the others. Over 80 per cent of our forms were from people in charge of local authority Homes and their information, therefore, dominates all total findings.

15. A total of 1,917 completed and usable forms referring to old people's Homes were returned—1,548 from local authority establishments, 232 from Homes run by voluntary organizations and 137 from those in charge of privately run establishments. This represents a response rate of 87 per cent for local authority Homes, 23 per cent for voluntary Homes and 10 per cent for private Homes.[1] We have therefore dealt with the three types separately throughout the section dealing with old people's Homes. As the response from private Homes was so small we have in a number of cases omitted tables dealing with them from this chapter, but the figures are available either in Appendix B or in the tables deposited with the National Council of Social Service or the National Institute for Social Work Training.

SUMMARY OF FINDINGS

RESIDENTS

i. The typical L.A. old people's Home contains between 16 and 50 clients, but there is an important minority of very large Homes with more than 250 clients. Voluntary, and even more so, private Homes tend to be smaller with a substantial majority containing 30 or fewer residents.

ii. Half of all residents are aged 80 or more and women outnumber men by 3 to 2. The preponderance of women is most marked in smaller L.A. Homes where they constitute two-thirds of all residents. In other words, men are relatively concentrated in very large Homes.

iii. The ratio of full-time care staff to residents is 1 to 6. In the L.A. Homes there are apparently no economies of size associated with the employment of full-time care staff.

STAFF

iv. Over four-fifths (82 per cent) of all care staff are full-time.

v. Two-thirds (65 per cent) of all care staff are non-resident. This is quite different from the findings for other residential Homes.

---

[1] The response rate from voluntary Homes appears to be low because we excluded the Homes run by caring staff under religious discipline (*see* Para. 2 above). It is difficult to estimate how many private Homes there are. We have assumed that in 1963 the same percentage of registered old people's homes were private Homes as are shown for 1960 in Professor Townsend's 'Last Refuge'.

vi. The employment of full-time resident staff is much more marked in smaller Homes and in voluntary and private Homes.

vii. Slightly over half of all resident care staff are aged 50 or more. The ratio of resident workers above this age is substantially higher in the smaller Homes (60 per cent).

vii. Over 80 per cent of resident care staff are women and nearly two-thirds are unmarried women.

ix. The average Home replaced one-fifth of its staff in the year preceding the survey.

x. At the time of the survey vacancies for care staff were equivalent to 4 per cent of total care staff.

xi. Nearly 40 per cent of Homes had had at least two heads in the preceding five years.

xii. A substantial majority of heads of Homes expressed themselves as completely satisfied with the accommodation provided for themselves and for their resident staff.

xiii. Practically all Homes were within 20 minutes walk of shops, cinemas, etc., and also had good access by public transport.

xiv. Over 80 per cent of all full-time care staff are without any formal qualifications for their work; the ratio of unqualified staff is much higher in L.A. Homes than in either voluntary or private Homes.

1. SIZE OF OLD PEOPLE'S HOMES

16. Homes have been grouped into six categories, according to the number of residents.

Table 4.1.
Size of Homes

No. of Residents	Local Authority %	Voluntary %	Private %
Under 16	4·7	8·6	34·3
16-30	33·7	50·4	40·2
31-50	38·0	31·0	21·1
51-100	17·0	6·5	2·9
101-250	5·3	3·5	1·5
Over 250	1·3	—	—
	100·0	100·0	100·0

17. This table shows that while one-third of L.A. Homes catered for small groups of under 30 residents, there were few very small Homes. The most usual size of Homes was for 31–50 residents. There still

remained a number of very large Homes for over 100 residents and although this was a small proportion of Homes, between them they contained a high proportion of old people—28 per cent.

18.   Of those voluntary organizations which completed the questionnaire, it seems that over 80 per cent are concerned with groups of between 16 to 50 old people.

19.   The private homes which replied are typically small; nearly three quarters of them have accommodation for 30 or less clients.

2. RESIDENTS (Q.6)

(a) *Local Authority Homes*

20.   The 1,548 L.A. Homes had at the time of the survey 71,833 people in residence—27,889 men and 43,944 women; i.e. the average Home contained 18 men and 28 women. This imbalance of the sexes was almost entirely due to the very high proportion of women aged 80 or more.

Table 4.2.
Age Composition of Residents in L.A. Homes

Age	Men %	Women %	Women as % of Men
Under 60	6	4	110
60–79	53	42	126
80 and over	41	54	207
	100	100	157

21.   The proportion of men to women varies with the size of the Homes; in the smaller Homes women outnumber men by almost 2 to 1, but in the very large Homes the two sexes are more nearly equal in number.

Table 4.3.
Sex Composition of Residents by Size of L.A. Home

Size of Home	Men %	Women %
30 or less	34	66 = 100 %
31–50	36	64
51–100	38	62
101 or more	45	55
All	39	61

22. The variation in sex composition between Homes of different sizes is apparently related to the fact that whereas an unusually high proportion of very old men (aged 80 and over) are in large Homes, very old women are concentrated in the smaller Homes.

Table 4.4.
Older Residents aged 80 and over distributed by size of L.A. Home

Size of Home	Men %	Women %	Ratio Women to Men
30 or less	18·4	20·2	2·3
31–50	31·9	35·2	2·3
51–100	22·3	23·4	2·2
101 or more	27·4	21·2	1·6
	100·0	100·0	2·1

(b) *Voluntary Homes*

23. The 232 voluntary Homes that replied had 7,321 residents—2,217 men and 5,104 women, i.e. the average Home contained almost 10 men and 22 women (a total of 32 as compared with 46 old people in the average L.A. Home). The ratio of women to men (2·3 to 1) is much higher than in L.A. Homes (1.6 to 1) and this imbalance is most marked among residents aged 80 and over.

Table 4.5.
Age Composition of Residents in Voluntary Homes

Age of Residents	Men %	Women %	Women as % of Men
Under 60	6	4	149
60–79	55	43	181
80 and over	39	53	322
Total	100	100	230

24. The proportion of men to women also varies with the size of the Homes. In the smaller Homes women outnumber men by over 5 to 1 but in the larger voluntary Homes (51 or more) the two sexes are almost equal in numbers.

Table 4.6.
Sex Composition of Residents by size of Home in Voluntary Homes

Size of Home	Men %	Women %
30 or less	18	82 = 100 %
31–50	31	69
51–100	34	66
101 or more	58	42
All	30	70

25. As in the L.A. Homes there is again a sex difference in the treatment of those aged 80 and over—men are relatively more concentrated in the larger Homes.

Table 4.7
Older Residents aged 80 and over distributed by size of Voluntary Home

Size	Men %	Women %	Ratio of Women to Men
30 or less	30	46	4·9
31–50	43	36	2·7
51 or more	27	18	2·1
Total	100	100	3·2

(c) *Private Homes*

26. Since there were only 137 completed forms from private Homes only the most tentative comments can be made about their figures. The average Home in our sample contained 4 men and 19 women, i.e. men constitute only 18 per cent of the residents in these Homes. Half the women were aged 80 or more, and the smaller Homes (i.e. 30 or less residents) housed slightly over half all residents in private Homes. There were, however, two Homes each with well over 100 residents and another 4 each with between 50 and 100 residents.

3   RATIO OF RESIDENTS TO STAFF

27. From Question 8 onwards a series of questions dealt with various aspects of staffing; before dealing with the replies in detail a crude summary of the numerical relations between care staff and residents is inserted here to give perspective to the subsequent discussion.

28. Part-time staff were converted into full-time equivalents and ratios of residents to full-time care staff were then calculated. The results are shown for each type of Home in Table 4.8. The ratio of residents to each member of care staff is lowest in L.A. Homes (6.1) and highest in voluntary Homes (7.4). This may partly be because voluntary Homes have a higher proportion of women residents, and women can perhaps look after themselves more easily than men can. Private Homes with an overall ratio of 6.7 came mid-way; this position, however, was entirely due to the very high resident/staff ratio in the private Homes with more than 100 residents. This extreme situation of understaffing was offset by another peculiarity of private Homes: in the smallest (under 16 clients) the resident/staff ratio is very low.

Table 4.8
Ratio of Residents to Full-time Care Staff, by size and type of Home

Residents	L.A.	Voluntary	Private	All Types
Under 16	5·6	6·1	3·3	4·8
16–30	6·8	7·0	7·0	6·9
31–50	6·7	8·0	7·6	6·9
51–100	6·2	6·8	6·3	6·2
101–250	5·4	8·3	18·7	5·6
251 or more	5·1	—	—	5·1
All	6·1	7·4	6·7	6·3

29. All three types of Home tend to show the same resident/staff ratios: they are lowest in the smallest Homes; they rise appreciably as the number of residents increase and then manpower diseconomies become significant for L.A. Homes when the number of residents exceed 100. In the voluntary and private Homes, however, increasing resident/staff ratios are associated with the very large Homes. It would be interesting to know why in L.A. Homes increases in size lead to a greater use of care staff in relation to residents. It is possible that this difference may be accounted for partly because a larger proportion of the more frail are cared for in the big L.A. Homes.

4. CARE STAFF (Q.8)
30. For the whole 1,917 Homes covered by the survey the composition of the care staff (14,494 persons) is as follows:

D

Table 4.9
Residence Composition of Care Staff

Full-time staff: resident in same building	29·6
resident in separate accommodation	3·6
non-resident	48·5
	81·7
Part-time staff: resident in same building	1·0
resident in separate accommodation	0·3
non-resident	17·0
Total	100·0

31. Two features stand out from these figures: for care staff the Homes depend overwhelmingly on full-time staff (82 per cent of all such employees), and a substantial majority of care staff (nearly 66 per cent) are completely non-resident—this holds true of both full-time and part-time care staff.

32. These general conclusions, however, have to be considerably modified when we look separately at type of Home and size of Home: broadly, private and voluntary Homes make much more use of full-time resident staff than do L.A. Homes, and smaller Homes, irrespective of sponsorship, similarly make much more use of full-time resident staff than do the large Homes.

(a) *Local Authority Homes*

Table 4.10
Residence Composition of Care Staff in L.A. Homes

No. of Residents	Full-time Staff				Part-time Staff			
	Res. same building	Res. separate	Non-resident	Total	Res. same building	Res. separate	Non-resident	
	%	%	%	%	%	%	%	
Under 16	61	2	16	79	4	1	16	= 100%
16–30	50	2	30	82	1	*	17	
31–50	35	2	41	78	1	*	21	
51–100	25	3	53	81	1	*	18	
101 and over	7	6	75	88	*	1	11	
All	27	3	52	82	1	*	17	

* less than 0·5 per cent.

33. The contrast between the small and large units is most acute; among the former roughly two-thirds of the staff are resident; in the largest Homes the proportion is as low as 14 per cent.

(b) *Voluntary Homes*

34. Because of the small numbers in the very small and very large voluntary Homes, we have grouped them into three size categories. Even so it is clear that the proportion of resident care staff falls with increasing size, but that even when size is held constant the voluntary Homes are staffed with a much higher proportion of resident care staff (61 per cent) compared with L.A. Homes (31 per cent).

Table 4.11
Residence Composition of Staff in Voluntary Homes

No. of Residents	Full-time Staff				Part-time Staff			
	Res. same building %	Res. separate %	Non-resident %	Total %	Res. same building %	Res. separate %	Non-resident %	
Under 31	62	3	14	79	2	*	19	= 100%
31–50	56	2	22	80	1	—	19	
51 and over	37	17	30	84	1	—	15	
All	54	6	21	81	1	*	18	

* less than 0·5 per cent.

(c) *Private Homes*

35. Private Homes follow voluntary Homes in employing a relative high proportion of resident care staff but are slightly more dependent than other types on part-time staff.

5. AGE COMPOSITION OF CARE STAFF (Q.10)

36. A majority of the care staff (54 per cent) is aged between 21 and 49; almost all the balance are aged 50 or more. There is, however, a significant difference between resident and non-resident staff; the latter are appreciably younger than the former.

Table 4.12
Age Composition of Care Staff

Age Group	Resident %	Non-Resident %	All %
Under 21	3	1	2
21–49	46	59	54
50 or over	51	40	44
Total	100	100	100

37. While type of Home makes very little difference to the age composition of staffs, size is a very different matter—especially in L.A.

Homes; the smaller Homes are staffed predominantly by people aged 50 or more while the larger Homes attract mainly younger people; the same is true of voluntary and private Homes.

Table 4.13
Age Composition of L.A. Homes Care Staff

No. of Residents	Age of Resident Staff				Age of Non-resident Staff			
	Under 21 %	21–49 %	50 and over %	Total %	Under 21 %	21–49 %	50 and over %	Total %
Under 16	—	39	61	100	—	60	40	100
16–30	1	41	58	100	1	53	46	100
31–50	2	46	52	100	1	50	39	100
51–100	3	51	44	100	1	59	39	100
100–250	2	58	41	100	2	55	43	100
251 and over	6	49	45	100	1	63	36	100
Total	2	47	51	100	1	59	40	100

6. SEX AND MARITAL STATUS OF RESIDENT CARE STAFF AND EMPLOYMENT OF THEIR SPOUSES (Q.11)

38. Slightly over one-third of all care staff (full-time and part-time) are resident either in the same building as the old people or in dwellings in the grounds of the Homes. Over 80 per cent of this resident care staff are women and nearly two-thirds are single women. Again there are substantial variations related to type and size of Homes. The proportion of women is highest in voluntary and private homes; this is largely because they employ single women and the L.A. Homes show a greater tendency to employ married couples.

Table 4.14
Sex and Marital Status of Resident Care Staff by Type of Home

	L.A. %	Voluntary %	Private %	All %
Married women:				
With husband working full-time in Home	15	7	10	14
With husband working part-time in Home	1	1	3	1
Husband not working in Home	5	5	9	5
Married men:				
With wife working full-time in Home	14	6	9	13
With wife working part-time in Home	1	*	—	1
Wife not working in Home	2	1	*	2
Single women	59	78	68	62
Single men	3	2	1	2
Total	100	100	100	100
Total women	80	91	90	82
Total men	20	9	10	18
	100	100	100	100

* less than 0·5 per cent.

39. The differences in staffing patterns arise almost entirely from the fact that while smaller L.A. Homes are similar to other Homes in their staffing arrangements, the large L.A. Homes depend much more on the engagement of married couples with both husband and wife working full-time.

Table 4.15
Sex and Marital Status of Resident Care Staff
L.A. Homes by Size of Home

	No. of Residents				
	Under 16 %	16–30 %	31–50 %	51–100 %	101 and over %
Married women:					
Husband working full-time in Home	11	11	15	20	17
Husband working part-time in Home	4	1	1	1	1
Husband not working in Home	7	4	6	4	4
Married men:					
Wife working full-time in Home	9	11	14	19	16
Wife working part-time in Home	—	*	1	1	1
Wife not working in Home	—	1	1	2	6
Single women	69	71	59	47	50
Single men	—	1	3	6	5
Total	100	100	100	100	100
Total women	91	87	81	72	71
Total men	9	13	19	28	29
	100	100	100	100	100

* less than 0·5 per cent.

7. STAFF WASTAGE AND REPLACEMENT

40. Continuity of care is very important to residents, so labour turnover was one of the factors we had to consider. To obtain a measure of staff turnover, heads of Homes were asked to state how many care staff had been appointed in the preceding twelve months, and how many had left. As the numbers for part-time staff were comparatively small, only the figures for full-time staff were analysed. The numbers of staff who were appointed as replacements have been expressed as a percentage of the total full-time care staff employed, and this gives the annual gains; the numbers of staff who left, given as a percentage of total staff employed, show the annual loss rate. Staff appointed to fill newly established posts, as a result of expansion, are shown separately at (b) below.

(a) *Gains and losses of full-time care staff, excluding heads of Homes* (Q.13a and Q.14)

41. The annual wastage of care staff for all old people's Homes replying was equal to one-quarter of total care staff employed. In voluntary Homes it was slightly higher, and in private Homes slightly lower, than in local authority Homes.

42. Losses were higher for non-resident than for resident staff in local authority Homes, but voluntary Homes had more losses among resident staff.

Table 4.16
Gains and Losses in full-time staff, over twelve months

Type of Home	Resident		Non-resident		Total	
	Gains	Losses	Gains	Losses	Gains	Losses
	%	%	%	%	%	%
L.A.	17	19	21	29	19	25
Voluntary	24	28	28	24	25	27
Private	25	23	18	23	23	23
Total	18	20	21	29	20	25

42. Over the period, staff replacements were fewer than losses, i.e., there was a decline in total staff. Moreover, this state of affairs emerged for practically all types and sizes of Homes, and for both resident and non-resident staff. Net loss was greatest among non-resident staff in local authority Homes; the failure to replace losses was most marked in the largest local authority Homes, for both resident and non-resident staff.

Table 4.17
Gains and Losses in Full-time Staff in L.A. Homes

No. of Residents	Resident		Non-resident	
	Gains	Losses	Gains	Losses
	%	%	%	%
Under 16	11	11	29	36
16–30	17	17	32	35
31–50	18	18	29	32
51–100	19	21	24	29
101 and over	8	20	13	26
Total	17	19	21	29

(b) *New Appointments* (Q.13b)

44. The whole sample reported only 394 appointments to new posts during the preceding twelve months; this was equivalent to a 3 per cent expansion in care staff; however, two-thirds of this growth occurred in L.A. Homes containing 31 to 100 residents and nearly three-quarters were non-resident posts. It would be rash on one year's figures to conclude that this is an established pattern of growth in the staffing of old people's Homes.

(c) *Vacancies* (Q.9)

45. At the time of the survey vacancies for care staff were equivalent to 4 per cent of total staff, and vacancies which had been unfilled for six months or more were equal to 1 per cent of all care staff. This seems very small, but when people have to be cared for staff have to be found somehow even if they are not always suitable; this may partly account for the high staff wastage.

(d) *Reasons for leaving* (Q.15)

46. Heads of Homes were asked to give for each person leaving in the preceding year the main reason for the departure, and the results were analysed. We became increasingly doubtful of the value of the replies as the analysis proceeded. First, because a substantial number of heads —over a quarter in the case of old people's Homes—did not give any reasons and, second, because one doubted whether staff gave an entirely frank reply on a written questionnaire, as experience indicates that quite other reasons emerge as one is enabled to probe deeper in face-to-face interviews. We have therefore not shown the results here, although the tables are available at the N.C.S.S. or the N.I.S.W.T.

(e) *Heads of Homes* (Q.16)

47. Among heads of Homes turnover is also on the high side. Nearly 40 per cent of all Homes had had at least two heads in the five years preceding the enquiry. This was highest in voluntary Homes—48 per cent.

48. In local authority Homes, the turnover of heads was most marked in the smaller Homes. This may be because heads move from a smaller to a larger Home, which up to now has been a form of promotion.

49. In voluntary Homes and in L.A. Homes it is in those of 31–50 residents that showed the smallest turnover of heads—two-thirds only had one head in five years.

Table 4.18
Turnover of Heads in Local Authority and Voluntary
Old People's Homes

	Number of Heads in preceding 5 years					
No. of residents	1		2		3 or more	
	L.A.	*Vol.*	*L.A.*	*Vol.*	*L.A.*	*Vol.*
	%	%	%	%	%	%
Under 30	57	47	30	33	13	20
31–50	67	62	26	18	7	20
51–100	62	29	31	42	7	29
101 and over	64	20	33	80	3	—
Total	62	50	29	30	9	18

8. VIEWS ON STAFF ACCOMMODATION (Q.17)

50. The assessment of the accommodation provided for care staff was made solely by heads of Homes who were asked to give their views on the accommodation provided for resident care staff. We could not ask all the staff for their opinion of their accommodation, so the heads of Homes gave their views of the accommodation provided for four types of staff shown separately—heads of Homes, married staff, single staff and for any students employed. Replies dealt with four main aspects of accommodation—privacy, space, heating and amenities (bathroom, lavatory, cooking and laundry facilities). Heads were asked to state whether each aspect was 'completely satisfactory', 'fairly satisfactory' or 'less than satisfactory'. We should perhaps explain why the question took this form. We wanted to know whether the accommodation provided for staff was adequate by modern standards, because we felt fairly certain this would be an important factor in recruiting suitable resident staff. Our original intention was to ask how many rooms they had, how big they were, how they were heated and so on. But the answers to these questions in our pilot surveys proved so detailed and diverse that we could not devise a form which would cover every kind of combination of accommodation which was in existence. So, as we really wanted to know whether staff were satisfied with the accommodation provided—no matter how good the providing authority thought it was, or if by our standards it was dingy and inadequate—what really mattered was whether the people in it were satisfied or not. So we asked heads of Homes to say whether they thought the various aspects of their own and their staff's provided accommodation was completely satisfactory and so on, or not.

(a) *Accommodation for Heads of Homes*

51. On every aspect a substantial majority of respondents described their own accommodation as completely satisfactory. These attitudes were usually more widespread among heads of local authority and voluntary Homes; the outstanding exception to this was that among heads of local authority Homes a large minority—41 per cent—were less than completely satisfied with the privacy of their quarters. Among heads of local authority Homes considerable dissatisfaction emerged on the provision of personal cooking facilities, also.

Table 4.19
'Completely Satisfactory' assessment of Accommodation

		Accommodation for Heads of Homes % Completely Satisfied	Accommodation for Married Staff % of Heads Completely Satisfied	Accommodation for Single Staff % of Heads Completely Satisfied
Privacy:	L.A.	59	67	56
	Voluntary	77	88	80
	Private	74	87	83
Space:	L.A.	73	86	60
	Voluntary	85	88	80
	Private	81	83	79
Heating:	L.A.	89	82	84
	Voluntary	94	100	92
	Private	86	87	91
Bathroom:	L.A.	84	82	68
	Voluntary	85	95	73
	Private	86	89	81
Lavatory:	L.A.	85	86	70
	Voluntary	86	92	78
	Private	84	87	84
Personal cooking facilities:	L.A.	59	67	38
	Voluntary	73	87	60
	Private	79	86	69
Personal laundry facilities:	L.A.	66	67	57
	Voluntary	80	88	77
	Private	85	90	82

(b) *Accommodation for other staff*

52. When they were asked to rate the accommodation provided for their married staff, the heads of homes were even more laudatory. At least 80 per cent of heads said almost every amenity was completely satisfactory. The only exceptions came from some L.A. Homes and related to privacy and facilities for personal cooking and personal laundry.

53. Heads of Homes' assessments of the accommodation provided for single staff was again highly favourable. The 'completely satisfactory' score was, however, consistently lower for L.A. Homes than for the other types and the shortcomings were most marked in L.A. Homes for privacy and facilities for personal cooking and personal laundry.

9. OTHER ACCOMMODATION AND AMENITIES FOR STAFF (Q.18)

(a) *Staff sitting-room for exclusive staff use*

54. Only 42 per cent of all Homes have a separate staff sitting-room. In L.A. Homes this provision is very much a function of size—the larger the Home the more likely it is to have a staff sitting-room. This, however, does not hold true to anything like the same extent for voluntary and private homes where even among the smallest units a majority claim to have a sitting-room set aside for exclusive staff use. As a result, the provision of separate staff sitting-rooms is much more common among private and voluntary Homes.

(b) *Multi-purpose staff sitting-room*

55. In over 30 per cent of Homes which responded there was a staff sitting-room which was not for the exclusive use of staff, but was used also for another purpose. There are no figures on this, but we saw staff sitting-rooms which were also used as a waiting room for visitors or an examination room, or an office. But again the incidence of such rooms is much lower in L.A. Homes (29 per cent) than in either voluntary Homes (42 per cent) or private Homes (37 per cent).

(c) *Separate staff dining-room*

56. Only 24 per cent of Homes have a separate staff dining-room. Again, these are much more frequently found in voluntary and private Homes, and again their incidence, especially in L.A. Homes, is a function of size—the larger the Home the more likely it is to have such a room.

(d) *Combined dining-room and sitting-room*

57. Slightly over 60 per cent of Homes have a combined dining-room and sitting-room; the proportion is lower in voluntary and private homes (53 per cent and 44 per cent respectively), and higher in L.A. Homes (63 per cent). Among the latter such a room is most commonly found in the middle sized Homes, with 74 per cent in Homes with 31 to 50 clients, and 69 per cent in Homes with 51 to 100 clients; between them these account for well over half all L.A. Homes.

(e) *Separate staff recreation room*

58. Only 3 per cent of all Homes have a separate staff recreation room. In L.A. Homes the proportion is even lower (2 per cent); practically all these are in the larger L.A. Homes, but even in those with over 100 residents the ratio is no more than 10 per cent.

(f) *Changing room for non-resident staff*

59. Less than half of all Homes (47 per cent) have a changing room for non-resident staff and its provision is largely determined by the size of the Home. Among the smallest (30 or fewer clients) roughly 25 per cent have a changing room, while in Homes with more than 100 residents the ratio is approximately 75 per cent.

(g) *Proximity to shops, cinemas etc.* (Q.19)

60. Over 90 per cent of Homes, irrespective of type and size, are located within a 20 minute walk of shops; and 62 per cent are within a 20 minute walk of cinemas, dance halls etc. This nearness to recreational facilities, however, is more common for private and voluntary homes where the ratio rises to 72 per cent (compared with 60 per cent for L.A. Homes).

(h) *Proximity to public transport*

61. Slightly over 80 per cent of all Homes, irrespective of type and size are on a bus route with services at least every half hour.

10. QUALIFICATIONS[1] OF CARE STAFF (Q.12)

(a) *Full-time staff*

62. Apparently 82 per cent of the full-time care staff were without any formal qualifications. This is an extremely disturbing figure. This proportion was even higher in L.A. Homes. By comparison, the smaller voluntary and private homes had staffs where larger pro-

[1] A full list of the qualifications asked for is set out in Appendix B 'Qualifications—description of terms'.

portions were qualified. Of those who were qualified, nearly all had nursing qualifications; only 2 per cent of full-time staff had taken the special 14-week course run by the N.O.P.W.C.

Table 4.20
Full-time Care Staff Qualifications
(i) *By type of Home*

	L.A. %	Vol. %	Private %
S.R.N.	7	19	23
S.E.N.	6	10	12
Domestic Science	*	1	2
University Degree	*	1	2
Soc. Science Diploma	*	*	1
N.O.P.W.C.	2	2	4
Other	1	2	4
None	85	67	59
Total**	101	102	107

* Less than 0·5 per cent.
** Totals add to more than 100 per cent because some members of staff had more than one qualification.

Table 4.21
Full-time Care Staff Qualifications
(ii) *By size of Home*
(L.A. and Voluntary Homes only)

No. of residents	Under 31		31–50		51–100		101 and over	
	L.A. %	Vol. %	L.A. %	Vol. %	L.A. %	Vol. %	L.A. %	Vol. %
S.R.N.	6	22	8	18	8	21	7	9
S.E.N.	9	10	7	11	6	8	5	7
Dom. Sci.	*	2	1	1	*	—	*	1
University degree	*	1	—	1	*	1	*	—
Soc. Sci. diploma	*	1	—	—	*	—	*	—
N.O.P.W.C.	3	2	3	4	1	1	*	—
Other	1	4	1	1	1	—	*	2
None	81	63	82	66	84	69	89	83
Total**	100	105	102	102	100	100	101	102

* Less than 0·5 per cent.
** Totals add to more than 100 per cent because some members of staff had more than one qualification.

63. When divided by size of Home, it appears that the larger the Home, the higher the proportion of unqualified staff; in the biggest L.A. Homes, as many as 9 out of 10 staff had no formal qualifications. Again, it is in the smaller Homes for less than 50 residents where there is the highest proportion of staff who had taken the N.O.P.W.C. 14-week course.

(b) *Part-time staff*

64. The sparsity of qualifications was even more marked among part-time client-care staff—89 per cent were without any formal qualifications of the kind listed on the questionnaire; of the 11 per cent with such qualifications, 6 per cent were S.R.N.'s, and 5 per cent S.E.N.'s. The proportions of qualified staff were much higher in voluntary and private Homes (31 per cent and 22 per cent respectively), and in L.A. Homes the proportions with qualifications were at their highest in the largest Homes.

II SURVEY OF CHILDREN'S HOMES

65. We received a total of 1,198 completed and usable forms, which represents about 64 per cent of all children's Homes. The majority of children's Homes—probably two-thirds—are run by local authorities, so we had far more returns for local authority Homes—950—than from establishments run by voluntary organizations—248.

66. The response rate for the two groups varied. 77 per cent of local authority Homes replied and 40 per cent of voluntary Homes.[1] For this reason, and because there are other important differences, the two types are shown separately throughout the section of the survey on children's Homes.

67. As 80 per cent of all questionnaires were from people in charge of L.A. Homes, their information dominates all total findings.

SUMMARY OF FINDINGS

RESIDENTS

i. L.A. Homes are smaller than those run by voluntary organizations. The average L.A. Home contained 13 children; the average voluntary Home contained 28.

ii. Boys outnumber girls by 3 to 2; the sexes are more equally balanced in the smallest Homes than in any others.

iii. The ratio of full-time care staff to children is 1 to 4. Staff ratios seems to bear little relation to size of Home or the age of the children

---

[1] The response rate from voluntary Homes appears to be low because we excluded the Homes with caring staff under religious discipline (*see* para. 2 above).

in care, except that in the largest voluntary Homes there are fewer staff in relation to the number of children than in the largest L.A. Homes.

STAFF

iv. Over four-fifths of all care staff are full-time.

v. Over four-fifths of all care staff are resident. This contrasts with the old people's field, where two thirds were non-resident.

vi. The employment of full-time resident staff is much more marked in the voluntary Homes than in L.A. Homes, especially in the smaller voluntary Homes.

vii. The age composition of resident care staff in children's Homes is appreciably younger than in old people's Homes. Only one-fifth, compared with one-half, were over 50 at the time of the survey. Voluntary Homes employed more young staff under 21 than L.A. Homes.

vii. 80 per cent of care staff are women, and nearly two-thirds of total staff are single women.

ix. The average Home replaced one-third of its staff in the year preceding the survey. This was higher than the figure for old people's Homes and Schools, and higher than for most of the other Homes.

x. At the time of the survey, vacancies for care staff were equivalent to 6 per cent of total care staff.

xi. Nearly 40 per cent of Homes had had at least two heads in the preceding five years.

xii. A substantial majority of heads of Homes expressed themselves as completely satisfied with the accommodation provided for themselves and their staff, but privacy was the least satisfactory aspect of their accommodation. A higher proportion of heads of voluntary Homes were completely satisfied with all aspects of accommodation than were heads of L.A. Homes.

xiii. Practically all Homes were within a 20-minute walk of shops, and had reasonably good access by bus to shops, cinemas and other recreational facilities.

xiv. 70 per cent of all full-time care staff are without any formal qualifications for their work; the ratio of unqualified staff is higher in L.A. Homes than voluntary Homes.

I. SIZE OF CHILDREN'S HOMES

68. Children's Homes have been grouped into five size categories.

The majority of L.A. Children's Homes—61 per cent—were small family group units of under ten children, and nine out of every ten L.A. children's Homes contained fewer than 20 children. In

Table 4.22
Size of Home

No. of Children	Local Authority %	Voluntary %
Under 10	61·0	7·7
11–20	28·5	45·2
21–50	8·3	35·9
51–100	1·7	6·1
Over 101	·5	5·1
	100·0	100·0

children's Homes run by voluntary organizations, there was not this emphasis on the small family group unit (less than 8 per cent). The most commonly found voluntary children's Home had 11–20 children, but a substantial number—over a third—had 21–50 children.

69. In contrast with the old people's field, for children it was the voluntary organizations which had the very large Homes. 25 per cent of the children in voluntary Homes were living in Homes of over 100 children (although in practice the children are probably cared for in smaller groups). In L.A. Homes only 10 per cent were in the very large Homes.

2. CHILDREN (Q.6)

70. The 1,198 Homes had at the time of the survey 19,133 children in residence—11,480 boys and 7,653 girls, i.e. the average children's Home contained 10 boys and 6 girls. But this conceals considerable variation. The average voluntary Home is more than twice as big—28 children—as the average L.A. Home—13 children.

Table 4.23.
Age Composition of Children by Size and Type of Home

	Local Authority			Voluntary		
	Under 5 %	5–14 %	15–20 %	Under 5 %	5–14 %	15–20 %
Under 10	7	86	7	8	72	20
11–20	8	83	9	17	77	6
21–50	16	76	8	12	80	8
51–100	12	82	6	21	69	10
101 and over	14	79	7	13	82	5
	10	82	8	15	78	7

71. The majority of children in residential care are between five and 15 but voluntary Homes have a higher proportion of children under five. This difference may be accounted for by the fact that Local Authorities may put more children under five in nurseries; the majority of nurseries from which we received replies were, in fact, Local Authority institutions.

72. In one size group—51–100—the voluntary Homes had a very large proportion of children under 5 (21 per cent). In the smallest size of voluntary Homes, there was a very big proportion of children over 15—20 per cent—whereas in all other Homes this older age group was not very significant.

73. There are three boys to every two girls in residential care. The variation in sex composition between various types of Homes is apparently related to the fact that the smallest family group Homes have the smallest proportion of boys in them; indeed the smallest voluntary Homes are the only category where there are fewer boys than girls. The disbalance between the sexes is most marked in local authority Homes of 11–50 children, and in voluntary Homes of 51–100 children.

Table 4.24
Sex Composition of Children by Size of Home

No. of children	Local Authority		Voluntary	
	Boys %	Girls %	Boys %	Girls %
Under 10	57	43	43	57
11–20	64	36	55	45
21–50	63	37	59	41
51–100	61	39	67	33
101 or more	59	41	61	39
All	60	40	60	40

3. RATIO OF CHILDREN TO CARE STAFF

74. From Question 8 onwards, as in the case of old people's Homes, a series of questions was asked which dealt with various aspects of staffing. Before dealing with the replies in detail, a crude summary of the numerical relations between care staff and children was made. Part-time staff were converted to full-time equivalents and the ratios of children to full-time care staff were then calculated. The results are shown for each type of Home.

75. There are about four children to every staff member, compared with an average of 6·3 in the old people's field. On the whole, the ratio

5. AGE COMPOSITION OF CARE STAFF (Q.10)

83. Two-thirds of the care staff (64 per cent) are aged between 21–49, 13 per cent are under 21 and 23 per cent are over 50. There is also a significant difference between resident and non-resident staff; resident staff are appreciably younger than non-resident staff. In old people's Homes it was non-resident staff who were younger.

Table 4.27
Age Composition of Care Staff

Age Group	Resident	Non-Resident	All
	%	%	%
Under 21	14	5	13
21–49	65	63	64
50 or over	21	32	23
Total	100	100	100

84. Different sizes of Homes show very different age composition. As might be expected, the smallest local authority Homes have very few staff under 21 (4 per cent) because in very small Homes the responsibility is considered too great for very young staff. But the very large children's Homes also employ very few junior staff (6 per cent). It is the middle-sized Homes of 21–50 children which employ most young staff (26 per cent). The propensity of the middle-sized L.A. Homes to attract younger care staff is mainly due to their employment of younger *resident* staff, but to a lesser extent it is also true of non-resident staff. It is the larger Homes which employ most resident care staff in the over 50 age group.

85. On the whole, voluntary Homes employ more young staff than local authority Homes—16 per cent of their resident staff are under 21; but only 10 per cent in L.A. Homes were under 21; 9 per cent of their non-resident staff were under 21; but only 5 per cent in L.A. Homes. In voluntary Homes the differences are less marked between the different sizes of Homes—the age composition of staff is not very different in the different size groups.

6. SEX AND MARITAL STATUS OF RESIDENT CLIENT-CARE
    STAFF AND EMPLOYMENT OF THEIR SPOUSES (Q.11)

86. 85 per cent of all care staff, full-time and part-time, are resident either in the same building as the children or in the dwellings in the grounds of the Home. 80 per cent of this resident care staff are women and 60 per cent are single women. This is particularly signifi-

cant in children's work, which has been generally considered to employ many more married couples than in the old people's field. Yet these figures show that the proportion of women and the proportion of unmarried women is the same in both fields. However, 1 in 5 of all staff in children's Homes is a man—nearly all of them married men.

87. Again, there are variations according to the type of Home. The proportion of women employed, and of single women, is much higher in the voluntary Homes, i.e. the local authority Homes show a greater propensity to employ married couples than the voluntary Homes do.

Table 4.28
Resident Care Staff by Type of Home

	Local Authority %	Voluntary %	All %
Married woman with husband employed full-time in Home	8	9	8
Married woman with husband employed part-time in Home	13	2	9
Married woman with husband not working in Home	4	1	3
Married man with wife employed full time in Home	20	11	17
Married man with wife employed part-time in Home	*	*	*
Married man with wife not working in Home	*	1	1
Single woman	53	72	60
Single man	2	4	2
Total	100	100	100
Total women	78	84	80
Total men	22	16	20
	100	100	100

* less than 0·5 per cent.

88. In local authority Homes the differences in staffing patterns arise from the fact that over half the smallest Homes are staffed by married couples either jointly employed full-time or with the wife full-time and the husband part-time (and presumably following his own job). This is a much higher proportion than for any other size of

Home. On the whole, the larger sized L.A. Homes employ the most single women. In the largest Homes of all, three out of four staff are single women. It is the small family group which is most likely to have a man on the staff, but even there, three out of four staff are women.

Table 4.29
Resident Care Staff by Size of Local Authority Homes

	Under 10 %	11–20 %	21–50 %	51–100 %	101 and Over %
Married women:					
With husband employed full-time in Home	2	14	13	9	3
With husband employed part-time in Home	24	7	1	7	9
With husband not working in the Home	7	3	1	3	2
Married men:					
With wife employed full-time in Home	26	20	13	15	8
With wife employed part-time in Home	*	1	—	—	—
With wife not working in the Home	*	—	1	1	*
Single women	41	54	69	62	74
Single men	*	1	2	3	4
Total	100	100	100	100	100
Total women	73	78	84	81	87
Total men	27	22	16	19	13
	100	100	100	100	100

Above "No. of Children" spans the five size columns.

* less than 0·5 per cent.

7. STAFF WASTAGE AND REPLACEMENT
(For methods of calculation, see para. 40 above.)

(a) *Gains and Losses of full-time care staff, excluding heads of Homes* (Q.13a and Q.14)

89. The annual wastage of full-time care staff for all children's Homes was 31 per cent. In view of the great importance of continuity for the care of children, this is a very disturbing figure. It is considerably higher than the wastage in old people's Homes—25 per cent.

90.   Our figures do not support the view which is sometimes expressed that staff of voluntary children's Homes leave less frequently than those in local authority Homes. Both show about the same proportion of losses—nearly one-third of resident staff every year, and even more non-resident staff.

91.   In local authority children's Homes, the smallest Homes showed much greater stability than average, and the two largest sizes of Homes showed very high losses—over 40 per cent of the resident staff had to be replaced each year, and two-thirds of the non-resident staff. On the whole, except for the largest Homes, annual losses slightly exceeded annual gains; i.e. there was a decline in total staff.

Table 4.30
Gains and Losses in Full-Time Staff in Local Authority Children's Homes

No. of children	Resident		Non-Resident		All Staff	
	Gains	Losses	Gains	Losses	Gains	Losses
	%	%	%	%	%	%
Under 10	15	17	35	42	17	18
11–20	28	35	38	31	29	34
21–50	32	37	18	21	28	33
51–100	43	41	67	79	46	46
101 and over	54	41	63	48	56	42
Total	28	30	38	37	29	31

92.   In voluntary Homes, the size of Home made comparatively little difference to turnover. The loss rate in Homes of 51–100 children was lower than average, but otherwise the different sizes of Homes, including the smallest, showed a very similar proportion of staff losses. However, voluntary Homes appear to have less difficulty in replacing staff than L.A. Homes. Over the year, gains and losses were equal for all full-time staff, and also for resident staff. In the case of non-resident staff, there was a substantial gain over the year.

(b) *New Appointments* (Q.13b)
93.   The whole sample reported only 111 appointments to new posts during the preceding twelve months; this was equivalent to a 2¼ per cent expansion in care staff. This expansion was almost entirely in the numbers of resident staff. It was fairly evenly divided between local authority Homes and voluntary Homes; the very smallest (under 10) and the largest (over 101) Homes accounted for very little of the

Table 4.31
Gains and Losses of Full-Time Staff in Voluntary Children's Homes

No. of children	Resident		Non-Resident		All Staff	
	Gains	Losses	Gains	Losses	Gains	Losses
	%	%	%	%	%	%
Under 10	31	33	*	—	33	33
11–20	29	31	25	—	29	30
21–50	32	31	82	64	33	32
51–100	22	23	39	39	23	17
101 and over	34	34	36	29	34	34
	30	30	48	38	31	31

* less than 0.5 per cent.

expansion. It would appear that two-thirds of the resident staff increases were in the three middle ranges of children's Homes. However, it would be rash to assume this was a pattern of growth in children's Homes on only one year's figures.

(c) *Vacancies* (Q.9)
94. At the time of the survey, vacancies for care staff were equivalent to 6 per cent of total staff, and vacancies that had been unfilled for six months or more were equal to 3 per cent of all care staff. This was higher than the proportion of unfilled vacancies in old people's Homes (4 per cent and 1 per cent respectively). Whilst we have no definite evidence, it is possible that authorities exercise greater caution in filling vacancies in children's Homes. In local authority children's Homes, the largest Homes showed a considerably higher proportion of vacancies (13 per cent) than did the smaller Homes, and 8 per cent of them had been unfilled for more than six months.

(d) *Reasons for leaving* (Q.15)
95. We have explained earlier (see above para. 46 in the survey of old people's Homes) our difficulties in tabulating reasons why staff left. The same difficulties apply to the survey of children's Homes, and we therefore do not give any figures, although they are available for consultation.

(e) *Heads of Homes* (Q.16)
96. The rate of resignation amongst heads of Homes is definitely on the high side. Nearly 40 per cent of Homes had had at least two heads in the five years preceding the enquiry. This was equally true of local authority and voluntary Homes: again there is no evidence from these

figures that staff stay longer in voluntary children's Homes—in fact in voluntary Homes of fewer than 10 children, well over a half (58 per cent) of the Homes had had more than one head in five years; this was the highest rate of turnover of all groups.

97.   Nor do the figures support the view that small children's Homes show greater stability than larger ones—in fact for both voluntary and local authority Homes, it is the larger Homes for over 50 children where fewer heads leave. This is particularly serious in the smallest Homes when the head of the Home is the housemother, perhaps with a husband, and they may be the only caring staff involved with the children. Yet in 1 in 10 of these smallest Homes there had been three or more changes in five years.

98.   However, the fact that about 60 per cent of heads of both L.A. and voluntary Homes had been in post for five years or more shows that heads of Homes stay in post longer than assistant staff.

Table 4.32
Turnover of Heads in Children's Homes

No. of Children	1 Head in 5 years		2 Heads in 5 years		3 or more	
	L.A.	Vol.	L.A.	Vol.	L.A.	Vol.
	%	%	%	%	%	%
Under 10	63	42	27	47	10	11
11–20	58	59	31	29	11	12
21–50	60	63	34	26	6	11
51 and over	71	68	29	29	—	3
Total	62	61	29	29	9	10

8. VIEWS ON STAFF ACCOMMODATION (Q.17)

99.   We have set out in the survey of old people's Homes (para. 50 above) the questions we asked about staff accommodation, and we have shown the proportion who said different aspects were completely satisfactory. We shall not repeat the Table for children's Homes because the pattern was broadly similar—most heads reported complete satisfaction. The detailed tables are available in the N.C.S.S. and N.I.S.W.T.

100.   There were some differences in reaction, however, compared with the replies from old people's Homes. They are as follows:

(a) Accommodation for heads of Homes

101.   On every aspect, a substantial majority of heads of Homes in voluntary Homes described their own accommodation as completely

satisfactory; but in local authority Homes, most heads did not consider the privacy of their quarters completely satisfactory and nearly half did not consider space completely satisfactory. A far larger proportion of heads of voluntary Homes were satisfied with their own accommodation in all its aspects than were heads of local authority Homes. In both types of Homes, a larger proportion were less than completely satisfied with privacy than with any other aspect.

(b) *Accommodation for married staff*

102. Heads of Homes were less enthusiastic about accommodation for married staff than the heads of old people's Homes. Again, a higher proportion of heads of voluntary Homes were completely satisfied than heads of local authority Homes. Privacy and space again were said to be the least satisfactory aspects of accommodation for married staff in local authority Homes—only half the heads of Homes thought they were completely satisfactory.

(c) *Accommodation for single staff*

103. On the whole, heads of Homes' assessments of the accommodation provided for single staff was favourable, but not so favourable as for their own accommodation. The 'completely satisfactory' score was again consistently lower in local authority Homes than in voluntary Homes, and for privacy the contrast was very marked—72 per cent of heads of voluntary Homes considered it was completely satisfactory; only 49 per cent in L.A. Homes thought it was.

(d) *Accommodation for students*

104. For students the same pattern of response is shown—two-thirds or more of heads of voluntary Homes said all aspects were completely satisfactory, but heads of L.A. Homes were not so satisfied, and privacy and to a lesser degree, space, were the two aspects where over 60 per cent of the heads of Homes said they were less than completely satisfied.

9. OTHER ACCOMMODATION AND AMENITIES FOR STAFF
(Q.18 and 19)
(a) *Staff Sitting-room for Exclusive Use*

105. Only 39 per cent of all Homes said they had a separate staff sitting-room. In larger local authority Homes this provision is rather a function of size—the larger the home the more likely it was to have a staff sitting-room. This is not true of voluntary Homes, where even amongst the smallest units a majority claim to have a sitting-room set

aside for exclusive staff use. As a result, the provision of separate staff sitting-rooms is twice as common in voluntary Homes.

(b) *Multi-purpose Staff Sitting-room*
106.   Over half (52 per cent) of Homes claimed to have a staff sitting-room which was used for other purposes. But the incidence of such rooms is slightly higher (53 per cent) in local authority Homes than in voluntary Homes (45 per cent).

(c) *Separate Staff Sitting-room*
107.   As would be expected in children's Homes, 95 per cent have no separate staff dining-room; staff and children eat together. Where separate provision existed, it was naturally more frequently to be found in the largest sized Homes. However, separate dining-rooms are much more frequently found in voluntary Homes (16 per cent) than in local authority Homes (3 per cent).

(d) *Combined Dining/Sitting-room*
108.   Very few children's Homes (13 per cent) have combined dining/sitting-rooms: the proportion is lower in local authority Homes (11 per cent) than voluntary Homes (21 per cent) and more frequent in large Homes than in small Homes.

(e) *Separate Staff Recreation Room*
109.   Only 2 per cent of all Homes have a separate staff recreation room, and practically all these are in the largest Homes.

(f) *Changing room for non-resident staff*
110.   Only 10 per cent have a changing room for non-resident staff; its provision is largely determined by the size of the Home, but 19 per cent of voluntary Homes have one, and only 7 per cent of local authority Homes.

(g) *Proximity to Shops, Cinemas*
111.   Over 90 per cent of Homes, irrespective of type and size are located within a 20 minute walk of shops and there is little difference between L.A. and voluntary Homes; 57 per cent are within a 20 minute walk of cinemas, dance halls, etc. This latter amenity is more common for voluntary Homes (66 per cent) than local authority Homes (54 per cent).
112.   85 per cent of all Homes, irrespective of size and type have shops and cinemas and other recreational facilities on a bus route with a service at least every half-hour.

10. QUALIFICATIONS OF CARE STAFF (Q.12)

(a) *Full-time staff*

113. Apparently 70 per cent of the care staff were without any formal qualifications at all. In voluntary Homes, a much smaller proportion (62 per cent) were entirely without qualifications than in local authority Homes (74 per cent). Only 18 per cent in all Homes were holders of the Residential Child Care Certificate or its equivalent (15 per cent holding the Certificate from the Central Training Council in Child Care or Scottish Advisory Council, 3 per cent holding a formal training qualification from a voluntary organization) which are the only training qualifications for work in residential children's Homes. In voluntary Homes nearly one-quarter of the staff (23 per cent) held one of these qualifications; in local authority Homes only 15 per cent did.

114. A further 5 per cent were trained nursery nurses, which is relevant in Homes with children under 5 years of age. A further 7 per cent had some form of nursing qualification, which is not necessarily

Table 4.33
Qualifications[1] of Full-Time Care Staff
(i) *By type of Home*

	Local Authority %	Voluntary %	All %
Certificate in Residential Child Care or equivalent from voluntary organization	15	23	18
N.N.E.B. or Nursery Warden	5	5	5
Nursing Qualifications	7	7	7
Certificate of Education	1	3	2
Domestic Science	1	1	1
Craft teaching qualification	*	1	1
University Degree	*	1	1
Social Science Diploma	*	1	
Other	*	1	1
None	74	62	70
Total**	103	105	106

* less than 0·5 per cent.
** Totals add to more than 100 per cent because some members of staff had more than one qualification.

[1] The full list of qualifications is set out in Appendix B.

relevant to the work in a children's Home, and there were a few staff with 'background' qualifications in domestic science, teaching or other forms of training.

115.   There was some variation in the supply of trained staff in Homes divided by size. In local authority Homes, the smaller the Home, the larger the proportion of staff with the Residential Child Care Certificate or its equivalent (19 per cent in the smallest Homes down to 9 per cent in the Homes for over 50 children).

Table 4.34
Qualifications of Full-time Care Staff
(ii) *By Size of Home*

No. of Children	Under 10		11–20		21–50		51 and over	
	L.A.	Vol.	L.A.	Vol.	L.A.	Vol.	L.A.	Vol.
	%	%	%	%	%	%	%	%
Cert. Residential Child-Care	18	19	17	10	10	21	8	17
Or equivalent	1	5	*	7	1	5	1	5
N.N.E.B. or Nursery Warden	4	5	5	4	7	5	5	6
Nursing Qualifications	7	7	5	7	8	5	6	7
Other, e.g. Dom. Science, Teaching, etc.	2	19	4	2	3	9	2	8
Total	32	55	31	30	29	45	22	43

* less than 0.5 per cent.

116.   It was only in the smallest voluntary Homes that more than half the staff had some kind of qualification (55 per cent); the medium Home of 11–20 children showed the smallest proportion of qualifications—only 30 per cent. In this size Home, only 17 per cent had the Child Care Certificate or its equivalent, whereas the smallest Homes had 24 per cent with this qualification, the Homes for 21–50 children had 26 per cent and Homes for 50 or more children 22 per cent.

(b) *Part-Time Staff*

117.   For part-time staff, the lack of training is even more marked. 91 per cent had no qualification at all; of the rest 3 per cent had nursing qualifications, 2 per cent were teachers, and only 1 per cent had the residential child care certificate or its equivalent. Voluntary Homes employed comparatively few part-time staff and therefore few conclusions could usefully be drawn, except that they appear to have a smaller proportion (75 per cent) of unqualified part-time staff than local authority Homes (94 per cent) and to have more staff with the Residential Child Certificate (3 per cent) than local authority Homes (1 per cent).

III. SURVEY OF OTHER RESIDENTIAL HOMES

Reception Homes, Hostels for working boys and girls, Nurseries for under-fives, Mother and Baby Homes, Homes for physically handicapped adults, Homes for mentally ill and mentally handicapped adults.

118. The questionnaires returned were divided into various categories for different types of Homes. We received 179 completed and usable forms from nurseries for children under five, 137 from reception Homes and centres, 122 from hostels for working boys and girls and 109 from mother and baby Homes. These numbers were not large enough to split by type of Home or size of Home, but they can be compared with the overall figures for children's Homes. We also received 81 completed questionnaires from Homes for physically handicapped adults and 58 questionnaires from Homes for mentally ill and mentally handicapped adults. These can be compared with the overall figures for old people's Homes.

119. The response rates for the different groups varied considerably. Our response rates for nurseries, reception Homes and hostels for adolescents was exceptionally high. In fact as a result of difficulties of definition we occasionally received two replies from the same institution. We can say that our figures covered the whole of the field in these categories. For mother and baby Homes, the response rate was 56 per cent; it was 32 per cent for physically handicapped adults and 20 per cent for mentally handicapped adults.

SUMMARY OF FINDINGS

RESIDENTS

i. The typical nursery contains 23 children; reception Homes have 20 children and hostels 12 children; all three have more boys than girls in them. The typical mother and baby Home has 13 girls in it; the typical Home for the physically handicapped has 40 residents; there are slightly more men than women in care in such Homes. Homes for the mentally handicapped have 19 residents; there are slightly more women than men in such Homes.

ii. Children in nurseries are nearly all under five but 5 per cent are over that age; in hostels for working boys and girls nearly all the children are 15–20, but 6 per cent are under 15 and 10 per cent are over 21. Reception centres have a comparatively high proportion (15 per cent) of children under five, but the majority of their children are of school age. Homes for physically handicapped adults have over one-third of their residents in the 60 plus age-group. Homes for mentally handicapped adults have one-fifth in the oldest age group. In mother and baby Homes, 73 per cent of the mothers or mothers to be are aged 15–20; and 3 per cent are under 15.

iii. Ratios of residents to full-time care staff varied with the type of resident from one to 1·5 in nurseries, one to 3·2 in reception Homes, one to 4.1 in mother and baby Homes, one to 4·3 in Homes for the physically handicapped, one to 4·8 in hostels and one to 6·3 in Homes for the mentally handicapped.

STAFF

iv. Over four-fifths of care staff in all types of Homes were full-time.

v. Between one-fifth and one quarter of care staff were non-resident in all types of Homes with two exceptions. In Hostels only 10 per cent were non-resident; in Homes for physically handicapped adults nearly two-thirds (62 per cent) of all care staff were non-resident.

vi. In nurseries over half the care staff were under 21; in other types of Homes a substantial proportion of staff were over 50, varying from the lowest—19 per cent in reception centres to the highest—42 per cent in mother and baby Homes.

vii. In nurseries and in mother and baby Homes, virtually all staff (98 per cent and 97 per cent) were single women, and in reception Homes nearly two-thirds were single women. One-third of the staff in hostels and the two kinds of Homes for handicapped adults were men and Homes for the mentally handicapped employed a high proportion of married staff—over two-thirds of total staff.

viii. The average Home replaced between a quarter and a third of its care staff in the year preceding the survey.

ix. At the time of the survey, vacancies for care staff were equivalent to between 5 per cent and 9 per cent of total staff in most types of Homes.

x. Heads of Homes showed the lowest turnover in Homes for the mentally handicapped (only one-third of these Homes had had more than one head in the preceding 5 years) and the highest in Homes for the physically handicapped (over half had had more than one head in five years).

xi. A substantial majority of heads of Homes expressed themselves as completely satisfied with the accommodation provided for themselves and their staff; but more of them were completely satisfied with their own accommodation than with that for their staff. Privacy, and to a lesser extent, space and personal cooking facilities were the aspects where a substantial proportion of heads were less than completely satisfied for themselves and for their staff.

xii. Practically all Homes were within a 20 minute walk of shops. Over two-thirds were within a 20 minute walk of cinemas and other recreation and over two-thirds were on a reasonably good bus service.

xiii. Over two-thirds of all full-time care staff were without any formal qualifications in all types of Homes except two. Of those qualified, in reception Homes and hostels most (16 per cent and 19 per cent) had residential child care qualifications; in Homes for the adult physically and mentally handicapped, most had nursing qualifications (33 per cent and 44 per cent). The two exceptions were mother and baby Homes, where only one-third of staff had no qualifications, and of those qualified, 29 per cent had nursery nurse or residential child care qualifications and 65 per cent had nursing qualifications; and nurseries where only half had no qualifications and of those qualified 36 per cent had nursery nurse qualifications and 12 per cent had nursing qualifications.

1. SIZE OF HOMES

120.   The average children's Home contained 16 children, (10 boys and 6 girls). Hostels for working boys and girls with 12 children (7 boys and 5 girls) were smaller on average and reception centres were on average larger with 20 children (11 boys and 9 girls). But the average nursery for under-fives was considerably bigger than ordinary children's Homes, with 23 children (14 boys and 9 girls).

121.   For mother and baby Homes, heads of Homes were asked to exclude the number of babies on the census date, and to return only the numbers of mothers or mothers-to-be in residence. The average number of girls in a mother and baby Home was 13, which means that the average mother and baby Home is small.

122.   Homes for physically handicapped adults were the biggest in this group with 40 residents. (21 men and 19 women.) This compares with an average of 46 residents in old people's Homes (18 men and 23 women). Homes for mentally ill and mentally sub-normal adults had 19 residents fairly evenly divided between the sexes (9 men and 10 women).

2. RESIDENTS (Q.6)

(a) *Sex composition*

123.   Reception Centres, Hostels and Nurseries shared a greater imbalance between the sexes than did the Homes for the two categories of handicapped adults.

Table 4.35
Sex composition for residents in other Homes

	Male %	Female %
Reception centres and Homes	56	44
Hostels for working boys and girls	57	43
Nurseries for under-fives	59	41
Mother and baby Homes	—	100*
Homes for physically handicapped adults	52	48
Homes for mentally handicapped adults	48	52

* Excluding babies.

(b) *Age composition*

124. Nearly all the children in nurseries are under five; nearly all the children in hostels for adolescents are over fifteen but one in twenty of the children in these two types of Homes is outside the age-group catered for. In reception Homes there is a higher proportion of children under five (15 per cent) than there are in ordinary children's Homes (11 per cent). In mother and baby Homes, three-quarters of the girls in care are between 15 and 20, but a substantial minority are over 21. 3 per cent of these unmarried mothers are under 15. In the Homes for physically handicapped adults over a third are aged 60 and over and in the Homes for mentally physically handicapped adults, one in five is over 60.

Table 4.36
Age composition of residents

Age of residents:	Under 5 %	5–14 %	15–20 %	21–59 %	60 and over %
Reception centres	15	77	8	—	—
Hostels for working boys and girls	—	6	84	10	—
Nurseries for under-fives	95	4	1	—	—
Mother and baby Homes	—	3	73	24	—
Homes for physically handicapped adults	—	*	11	51	38
Homes for mentally handicapped adults	—	*	12	66	22

3. RATIO OF RESIDENTS TO STAFF

125. Part-time staff were converted to full-time equivalents and the ratios of residents to full-time care staff were then calculated. The results are shown for each type of Home.

Table 4.37
Ratio of Residents to each full-time equivalent care staff

Reception Homes	3·2
Hostels for working boys and girls	4·8
Nurseries for under-fives	1·5
Mother and baby Homes	4·1
Homes for physically handicapped adults	4·3
Homes for mentally handicapped adults	6·3

126. As might be expected, reception Homes have more staff in relation to children (3·2) than do ordinary children's homes (3·9) and hostels for adolescents have fewer staff, although even they have one member of staff for fewer than 5 children. In nurseries for babies and very young children, the staff ratio of one to 1·5, which seems high, is considerably below the recommended ratio of one to 1·2, but this does not appear to be due to an excessive number of unfilled vacancies —in fact nurseries have fewer vacancies than other children's Homes (see paragraph 146 below).

127. Mother and baby Homes and Homes for physically handicapped adults have ratios of 4·1 and 4·3 residents to each staff member. Homes for mentally handicapped adults have a ratio of residents to staff of 6·3 which is the same as the figure for old people's Homes.

4. CARE STAFF (Q.8)

128. For the Homes covered, the composition of the care staff (902 in reception Homes, 346 in hostels, 2,821 in nurseries, 371 in mother and baby Homes, 841 in Homes for physically handicapped adults and 185 in Homes for mentally handicapped adults), was as follows:

Table 4.38

	Reception Homes %	Hostels %	Nurseries %	Mother and Baby Homes %	Phys. Hand. Adults %	Ment. Hand. Adults %
Full-time Staff						
Resident in same building	72·7	79·0	62·1	67·3	31·5	66·0
Resident in sep. acc.	4·3	1·4	14·1	3·2	6·0	2·2
Non-resident	11·7	2·0	17·5	15·3	43·2	19·4
	88·7	82·4	93·7	85·8	80·7	87·6
Part-time Staff						
Resident in same building	2·0	8·7	·4	·8	·2	3·8
Resident in sep. acc.	·3	·8	·1	·5	·4	—
Non-resident	9·0	8·1	5·8	12·9	18·7	8·6
Total	100·0	100·0	100·0	100·0	100·0	100·0

129. Like other residential Homes, these types of Homes depend overwhelmingly on full-time staff—over 80 per cent in all cases, and 94 per cent in the case of nurseries. They also depend on resident staff, but not to the same extent. With one exception, over 70 per cent of all staff were resident in the same building or within the grounds of the establishment. It is perhaps surprising that amongst this group, it is hostels for adolescents which have the lowest proportion of non-resident staff.

130. The exception to the general pattern in this group are the Homes for physically handicapped adults, where 62 per cent of the staff are non-resident. This is similar to old people's Homes, where 66 per cent are non-resident.

5. AGE COMPOSITION OF CARE STAFF (Q.10)

131. Two-thirds of the care staff in reception Homes are aged 21–49. Amongst resident staff the rest are fairly evenly divided between those under 21 and those over 50; amongst non-resident staff, the majority of the balance are over 50. The age distribution in reception centres is very similar to that in ordinary children's Homes, but ordinary children's Homes showed a slightly higher proportion over 50—23 per cent—than did reception centres—19 per cent.

132. In hostels for working boys, two-thirds of the staff are 21–49, and almost all the rest are over 50. The proportion of young staff under 21 employed is very small—2 per cent. This group has a staff structure very much more like old poeple's Homes than the other children's Homes.

133. In nurseries, as might be expected, more than half the staff (54 per cent) is under 21, and this is almost entirely due to the employment of very young *resident* staff. The rest of the staff are in the middle age-group, 21–49; very few resident staff in nurseries are over 50. Non-resident staff showed somewhat higher proportions in the older age-groups, but even here a quarter of the staff were under 21. This preponderance of young staff is probably partly accounted for by the presence of young girls who are student nursery nurses. We know that a high proportion of the staff have nursery nurse qualifications (see Table 4.43 below).

134. In mother and baby Homes, very few staff are under 21 (4 per cent); nearly half (42 per cent) are over 50. Non-resident staff tend to be younger than resident staff.

135. The two types of Homes for handicapped adults have 60 per cent or more of their staff in the 21–49 age-group. They employ very few under 21, and over a third—36 per cent—are aged 50 or over. This

is a smaller proportion than in old people's Homes, where 44 per cent of staff were 50 or over.

Table 4.39
Age Composition of Care Staff
(i) *Reception Homes and Centres*

Age-Group	Resident %	Non-Resident %	All %
Under 21	14	7	13
21–49	69	64	68
50 and over	17	29	19
Total	100	100	100

(ii) *Hostels for Working Boys and Girls*

Age-Group	Resident %	Non-Resident %	All %
Under 21	2	3	2
21–49	64	62	64
50 and over	34	35	34
Total	100	100	100

(iii) *Nurseries for Children under Five*

Age-Group	Resident %	Non-Resident %	All %
Under 21	63	24	54
21–49	32	64	39
50 and over	5	12	7
Total	100	100	100

(iv) *Mother and Baby Homes*

Age-Group	Resident %	Non-Resident %	All %
Under 21	5	2	4
21–49	49	65	54
50 and over	46	33	42
Total	100	100	100

(v) *Homes for physically handicapped Adults*

Age-Group	Resident	Non-Resident	All
	%	%	%
Under 21	5	2	3
21–49	62	60	61
50 and over	33	38	36
Total	100	100	100

(vi) *Homes for mentally handicapped Adults*

Age-Group	Resident	Non-Resident	All
	%	%	%
Under 21	1	—	1
21–49	66	56	63
50 and over	33	44	36
Total	100	100	100

6. SEX AND MARITAL STATUS OF RESIDENT CARE
STAFF AND EMPLOYMENT OF THEIR SPOUSES (Q.11)

136. In ordinary children's Homes, 76 per cent of all full-time care staff were resident, either in the same accommodation or in separate accommodation within the grounds. 80 per cent of this resident care staff were women and nearly two-thirds were single women. Reception Centres broadly follow the same pattern but the other types of children's Homes are different.

137. An unusual feature of the children's field is to be found in hostels for adolescents. As over one-third of their staff is male and the majority are married men with wives who were also working in the hostel, there is a much smaller proportion of single women than in any other group caring for children in residence.

138. On the other hand, nurseries and also mother and baby Homes depend almost entirely on single women—98 per cent and 97 per cent respectively of the total staff. As far as nurseries are concerned, as two-thirds of their resident staff are under 21, this preponderance of single women is perhaps to be expected. But in mother and baby Homes where the work would appear to be particularly suitable for married women and there is some evidence that the girls prefer married matrons, it seems surprising that virtually no married women are employed. A high proportion of these unmarried women staff (42 per cent) are over 50. It seems very unlikely that single women in these proportions will be available to replace them when they retire.

139. In the Homes for physically handicapped adults, a third of the staff are men, half of them married and half single. Most of the women employed are unmarried.

140. Homes for mentally handicapped adults are unusual in that most of the staff are married (36 per cent are married women and 32 per cent are married men). This is the only type of Home where only a quarter of the staff are single women.

Table 4.40
Resident Care Staff by Sex and Marital Status

	Reception Homes %	Hostels %	Nurseries %	Mother and Baby Homes %	Phys. Hand. Adults %	Ment. Hand. Adults %
Married women with husband employed full-time in Home	11	17	*	—	8	26
Married women with husband employed part-time in Home	3	7	*	1	1	5
Husband not working in Home	3	2	1	2	4	5
Married men, with wife employed full-time in Home	13	25	*	—	9	29
Married men, with wife employed part-time in Home	1	1	*	—	1	*
Wife not working in Home	1	1	—	—	7	3
Single women	63	37	98	97	54	25
Single men	5	10	1	*	16	7
Total	100	100	100	100	100	100
Total women	80	63	99	100	67	61
Total men	20	37	1	*	33	39
	100	100	100	100	100	100

* less than 0·5 per cent.

7. STAFF WASTAGE AND REPLACEMENT

141. For methods of calculation, see survey of old people's Homes, para. 40 above.

(a) *Gains and losses of full-time care staff, excluding heads of Homes* (Q.13a and Q.14)

142. For the Homes here under discussion, all types had to replace at least a quarter of their staff every year. Staff losses ranged from 25 per cent for hostels for adolescents and Homes for the mentally handicapped to 39 per cent for nurseries—a very high figure. This compares

with staff turnover of 31 per cent in children's Homes and of 25 per cent in old people's Houses.

143. For reception Homes and nurseries, Homes for physically handicapped adults and Homes for mentally handicapped adults, losses of resident staff were higher than for non-resident staff.

Table 4.41
Gains and Losses in Full-time Staff (excluding the Head of the Home)
over Twelve Months

	Resident		Non-resident		All Staff	
	Gains	Losses	Gains	Losses	Gains	Losses
	%	%	%	%	%	%
Reception Homes and centres	34	37	29	27	33	36
Hostels for working boys and girls	24	24	100	86	26	25
Nurseries for under-fives	39	41	32	31	36	39
Mother and baby Homes	25	25	35	40	27	28
Homes for physically handicapped adults	33	37	28	27	30	32
Homes for mentally handicapped adults	20	25	47	22	26	25

144. Hostels for working boys and girls showed gains and losses fairly evenly balanced, but nurseries and reception Homes showed that over the year there were more losses than gains amongst their resident staff, i.e. a decline in total resident staff, which for these two categories was a high proportion of all their staff. (77 per cent and 79 per cent staff were resident.) In non-resident staff for these two categories, gains exceeded losses. Mother and baby Homes showed replacements equalling losses for resident staff, but more losses than gains in non-resident staff. Homes for physically handicapped adults showed more losses than gains for resident staff but an almost equal balance for non-resident staff. Homes for mentally handicapped adults showed more losses than gains for resident staff, but nearly twice as many gains as losses for non-resident staff, which are numerically important in this type of Home.

(b) *New appointments* (Q.13b)

145. Heads of Homes were asked to say how many staff had been appointed to fill new posts. Reception Homes reported 22 appointments to new posts during the preceding twelve months; this was equivalent to a 3 per cent expansion of client-care staff. Hostels reported 12 appointments, a 5 per cent expansion of staff, and nurseries appointed 27 to new posts, a 1 per cent expansion. Mother and baby Homes reported 5 new appointments, a 2 per cent expansion and Homes for the mentally handicapped had 18 new appointments, an

11 per cent expansion. In all five types of Homes the majority of new appointments were to residential posts. But in Homes for physically handicapped adults, of the 35 new appointments (a 5 per cent expansion) the majority—23 new posts—were for non-resident staff.

(c) *Vacancies* (Q.9)

146. At the time of the survey, vacancies for care staff were equivalent to 8 per cent of total staff for reception Homes and hostels for adolescents, and 5 per cent for nurseries. Vacancies which had been unfilled for more than 6 months were 2 per cent for nurseries and reception Homes and 3 per cent for hostels. In Mother and baby Homes, there were vacancies equivalent to 7 per cent of total staff, 5 per cent of them of long standing. In Homes for the physically handicapped vacancies were equal to 5 per cent of total staff, but only 1 per cent were of long standing. In Homes for the mentally handicapped, vacancies were high—equivalent to 9 per cent of total staff— the highest in any type of home except girls approved schools, and 3 per cent had been unfilled for more than six months.

(d) *Reasons for leaving* (Q.15)

147. We have explained earlier our difficulties in tabulating the reasons given when staff left. (See survey of old people's Homes, para. 46 above.)

(e) *Heads of Homes* (Q.16)

148. Among heads of Homes, turnover is on the high side. Just over 40 per cent of hostels for adolescents and nurseries had had more than one head in the preceding five years—the same figure as for ordinary children's Homes. Heads of Homes for the physically handicapped showed greater turnover than any other kind of Home. Over half these Homes had had more than one head in five years (53 per cent). For reception Homes and mother and baby Homes very nearly half (48 per cent and 46 per cent) had had more than one head over the period. As reception Homes take children for comparatively short periods, possibly this rate of turnover matters less in their case than in other types of establishments.

149. However, it must be noted that in mother and baby Homes and in Homes for the physically handicapped, one in every five Homes had had three or more heads in five years.

150. Heads of Homes for the mentally handicapped showed more stability than any other type of Home. Two-thirds of the heads had been in post for more than five years.

Table 4.42
Turnover of Heads of Homes

	Number of Heads in preceding five years			
	1	2	3 or more	Total
	%	%	%	%
Reception Homes	52	39	9	100
Hostels for working boys and girls	59	30	11	100
Nurseries	58	28	14	100
Mother and baby Homes	54	26	20	100
Physically handicapped adults	47	31	22	100
Mentally handicapped adults	66	22	12	100

8. VIEWS ON STAFF ACCOMMODATION (Q.17)

151. In the survey of old people's Homes (see para 50 above) we have explained our questions on accommodation. The views expressed by the heads of these Homes about accommodation are very similar to those in the larger categories. We therefore do not give individual tables, but the main points of difference are here emphasized.

152. On balance, more heads of Homes expressed themselves as completely satisfied with their own accommodation than they did for their staff's accommodation, especially for single staff. This is the opposite of what we found for old people's Homes.

153. On the whole, a higher proportion of the heads of the two types of Homes for handicapped adults said accommodation for themselves and their staff was completely satisfactory than did the heads of the other Homes.

(a) *Accommodation for Heads of Homes*

154. On every aspect, a majority of the heads of Homes described their own accommodation as completely satisfactory; but a larger proportion were less than completely satisfied with the privacy of their accommodation than any other aspect. A substantial minority of heads of reception centres were less than completely satisfied with the space provided for them, and a sizable minority of heads of reception Homes, mother and baby Homes and nurseries said they considered their personal cooking facilities were less than completely satisfactory.

(b) *Accommodation for other staff*

155. The views of heads of Homes on the accommodation provided for their married staff followed very much the same pattern as their views on their own accommodation. A majority said all aspects were completely satisfactory, but privacy was the aspect with which a

substantial minority were less than completely satisfied. Half of the heads of reception centres said space and personal cooking facilities were less than completely satisfactory.

156. Nearly all the mother and baby Homes said accommodation for married staff was completely satisfactory in every aspect but as very few staff in these Homes are married (3 per cent) these replies are based on very few respondents.

157. For single staff, heads expressed themselves as less satisfied than they had been for their own accommodation. Again, privacy was the least satisfactory aspect.

158. A higher proportion of the heads of reception centres and nurseries were less than completely satisfied with space provided for their single staff than the heads of all the other types of Homes.

159. More than half the heads of reception centres and heads of Homes for the mentally handicapped were less than completely satisfied with the personal cooking facilities available for their single staff.

9. OTHER ACCOMMODATION AND AMENITIES FOR STAFF

(a) *Other Staff Rooms* (Q.18)

160. Of nurseries, Homes for the physically handicapped and reception centres, about two-thirds reported they had a staff sitting-room for exclusive staff use, whereas only about half the Hostels for working boys and girls, mother and baby Homes and Homes for the mentally handicapped said they had. 59 per cent of mother and baby Homes, 44 per cent of nurseries, 42 per cent of reception Homes and 37 per cent of hostels and Homes for the mentally handicapped said that staff sitting-rooms were used for other purposes as well, but only 34 per cent of Homes for the physically handicapped.

161. Half the nurseries had a separate staff dining-room, and half did not. Nearly all the mother and baby Homes, reception Homes and Hostels (90 per cent, 92 per cent and 95 per cent) did not have a separate staff dining-room, presumably because the staff ate with the children or residents. 38 per cent of Homes for the physically handicapped and 24 per cent of those for the mentally handicapped had a separate staff dining-room. Half the nurseries and Homes for the physically handicapped and those for the mentally handicapped had a combined dining and sitting-room; only about one-fifth of the reception Homes and the hostels and 38 per cent of the mother and baby Homes had a combined dining/sitting-room.

162. In all types of Homes, over 90 per cent had no separate staff recreation room. Not surprisingly, nurseries, which employ more staff

than any other type of Home in this group, more frequently said they had this separate staff recreation room.

163.   Over 70 per cent of the first three types of Homes had no changing room for non-resident staff, but for the last three, over 50 per cent said they had such a room.

(b) *Proximity to the shops, cinemas etc.* (Q.19)

164.   Nearly all Homes were within 20 minute walk of shops—94 per cent of reception Homes, 89 per cent of nurseries, 97 per cent of mother and baby Homes, 74 per cent of Homes for the physically handicapped and 100 per cent of hostels and Homes for the mentally handicapped: and over two-thirds of most types were within 20 minutes walk of cinemas and other recreational facilities. The only exception was Homes for the physically handicapped (56 per cent).

165.   Over two-thirds of all types of Homes were on a reasonably good bus service for both shopping and recreation. In the case of mother and baby Homes and Homes for the mentally handicapped, and hostels for working boys and girls, over 90 per cent were.

10. QUALIFICATIONS[1] OF CARE STAFF (Q.12)

(a) *Full-Time Staff*

166.   Nurseries for children under-five are the only kind of residential establishment in which as many as half the staff hold a formal qualification relevant to the work they were doing; 36 per cent of all staff hold a nursery nurse's or nursery warden's certificate. In reception Homes, the pattern is broadly similar to that of qualified and unqualified staff in ordinary children's Homes. Two-thirds of the staff held no qualifications at all.

167.   Hostels for working boys and girls showed an even larger proportion of staff—77 per cent—without formal qualifications, more than any other kind of residential Home for children. Those with qualifications had nearly all taken the residential child-care training.

168.   Mother and baby Homes have a very much smaller proportion of untrained staff—only 34 per cent—than any other type of residential Home. Of those that had taken training almost all had a nursing qualification, 65 per cent (of these 32 per cent were state registered nurses and 26 per cent state certified midwives, some staff no doubt holding both qualifications). This is by far the largest proportion of nurses employed in any type of Home. 11 per cent of the other

[1] A full list of qualifications is set out in Appendix B.

qualified staff had nursery nurse training, and 18 per cent held the Residential Child Care certificate or its equivalent.

169. In Homes for physically handicapped adults, 65 per cent had no qualifications, 33 per cent of staff had nursing qualifications and a small proportion held other qualifications.

170. In Homes for mentally handicapped adults, three-quarters had no formal qualification. 44 per cent had nursing qualifications and 4 per cent had taken the residential child care training.

Table 4.43
Qualifications of Full-time Care Staff

	Reception Homes %	Hostels for working boys and girls %	Nurseries for under-fives %	Mother and baby Homes %	Homes for phys. hand. adults %	Homes for ment. hand. adults %
Cert. Residential Child Care or equiv. from vol. org.	16	19	4	18	2	4
N.N.E.B. or Nursery Warden	7	—	36	11	*	—
Nursing qualifications	8	5	12	65	33	44
Certificate of Education	2	2	2	3	2	1
Domestic Science qualification	1	3	*	3	1	2
Craft Teaching tech. qualif.	1	2	*	1	3	1
University degree	1	1	—	1	*	1
Social Science Diploma	1	1	*	*	*	—
Other	1	1	1	2	3	2
None	66	77	52	34	65	76
Total‡	104	111	107	138	109	131

* less than 0·5 per cent.

‡ Totals add to more than 100 because some members of staff have more than one qualification.

(b) Part-time Staff

171. In nurseries over a quarter of the part-time staff had relevant qualifications for the work they were doing. 12 per cent had trained as nursery nurses, 4 per cent as residential child care workers, and 11 per cent had nursing qualifications; a further 3 per cent had background qualifications. But even so, 72 per cent had no formal qualifications at all.

172. In reception Homes, 82 per cent of the part-time care staff had no qualifications. 8 per cent had taken nursing training and 6 per cent had some teaching qualifications. 4 per cent had other qualifications.

173. In hostels for working boys and girls, 85 per cent of the part-time staff had no formal qualifications; 5 per cent had taken the residential child care certificate; 7 per cent had had nursing training and 4 per cent had other qualifications.

174. In mother and baby Homes, half the part-time staff had no qualifications and nearly all the trained staff had nursing qualifications. Similarly, in the two types of Homes for handicapped adults, three-quarters or more of the part-time staff had no training, and nearly all those who were trained had nursing qualifications.

IV. SURVEY OF APPROVED SCHOOLS, REMAND HOMES AND SPECIAL SCHOOLS

175. A total of 542 completed and usable forms were returned from these establishments in the U.K.—89 from Approved schools, 54 from remand Homes and 399 from special schools. This represents a high response rate from two of these groups—83 per cent of remand Homes and 91 per cent of special schools, and quite a good response from approved schools—59 per cent.

176. We have not further divided these schools and Homes by type (local authority owned or voluntary owned) or size, as it seemed to be of more significance to staffing problems to divide the schools according to the kind of children being cared for. The approved schools[1] in most tables are split into three groups—boys' junior and intermediate schools; boys' senior schools; girls' approved schools. Special schools are divided into six categories—for the blind and partially blind; for the deaf and partially deaf; for the physically handicapped; for the educationally sub-normal; for maladjusted children; and other schools[2].

SUMMARY OF FINDINGS

CHILDREN

i. Approved Schools for boys, whether Junior and Intermediate or senior, have an average size (92 boys) three times as great as either Approved Schools for girls or Remand Homes. Among the Special Schools, those for the maladjusted contain a small average number of children (25); those for the mentally sub-normal and the physically handicapped contain more than twice as many, and those for the blind and for the deaf have four times as many children.

ii. The Approved Schools and Remand Homes covered by the survey contained 7,206 boys and 982 girls. The ratio of boys to girls was higher for the Approved Schools (7·7 to 1) than for the Remand Homes

---

[1] Classifying schools have been excluded from the returns.
[2] Other schools include schools for epileptic children, those suffering from speech defects, and those suffering from more than one handicap. Schools for delicate children are included with schools for the physically handicapped.

(6 to 1). The girls were fairly evenly divided between two age groups, under 15 and 16 to 20, but a large majority of the boys were in the younger group. At the Junior and Intermediate Approved Schools one boy in every six was aged 16 to 20, and at the Senior Schools one boy in every seven was aged 5 to 15.

iii. The Special Boarding Schools contained 22,238 children, the great majority of whom were resident, but at schools for the deaf one in five attended daily, and at schools for the educationally sub-normal one in ten did so. The ratio of boys to girls was 1·7 to 1 overall, but at schools and homes for the maladjusted boys outnumbered girls by 4 to 1. 92 per cent of the children were aged from 5 to 15.

iv. In Approved Schools and Remand Homes the ratio of residents to full-time care staff rises as the average number of residents increased—3·1 to 1 at Remand Homes, 4·1 to 1 at Approved Schools for girls, and 10·3 to 1 at Approved Schools for boys. In Special Schools the type of disability also affects the resident to staff ratio, which is 4·1 to 1 in schools for the physically handicapped, 6 to 1 in those for the maladjusted, 7·9 to 1 in those for the educationally sub-normal and for the deaf, and 9·1 to 1 in those for the blind.

STAFF

v. Over five-sixths of all care staff are full-time (92 per cent in Approved Schools, 89 per cent in Remand Homes, 86 per cent in Special Schools).

vi. Nearly two-thirds (63 per cent) of the care staff in Special Schools are resident in the same building as the children, and half the care staff at Approved Schools and Remand Homes.

vii. The proportion of full-time care staff resident in the same building is much higher in Approved Schools for girls than in Approved Schools for boys or in Remand Homes, and is much lower in schools for the physically handicapped than in the other Special Schools.

viii. The proportion of care staff, both full-time and part-time, who are resident either in the school or in separate accommodation in the grounds and outside, ranges from 83 per cent at Approved Schools and 74 per cent at Special Schools to 59 per cent at Remand Homes.

ix. More than two-thirds (68 per cent) of the care staff at Approved Schools and Remand Homes are aged from 21 to 49, and almost all the remainder are older than this. The proportion of older staff is greater at Junior and Intermediate Approved Schools for boys than at those for senior boys.

x. A quarter of the care staff at Special Schools are aged 50 or over, and a sixth are under 21. The employment of very young care staff is most marked at schools for the physically handicapped and least marked at schools for the maladjusted.

xi. Three-quarters of the resident care staff at Special Schools are women and two-thirds are single women. Schools for the blind and for the deaf mainly employ single women. Schools for the maladjusted depend much more on married couples with both husband and wife working full time. 90 per cent of the resident care staff at Approved Schools for girls are single women. Approved Schools for senior boys employ a higher percentage of married men (58 per cent) than those for younger boys (39 per cent), and a lower percentage of women (27 per cent compared with 37 per cent). At Remand Homes, where the ratio of boys to girls is 6 to 1, two-fifths of the resident staff are women and half of these are single.

xii. The average school replaced almost a quarter of its full-time care staff in the year preceding the survey.

xiii. At the time of the survey, vacancies for care staff at Approved Schools for girls were equivalent to 15 per cent of total care staff. The position was better at Approved Schools for senior boys (8 per cent), Remand Homes (7 per cent), and at Junior and Intermediate Schools for boys and at the Special Schools (5 per cent).

xiv. 27 per cent of schools and homes had had at least two heads in the preceding five years. This is considerably lower than in most residential Homes.

xv. The majority of heads of Approved Schools and Special Schools expressed themselves as completely satisfied with accommodation provided for themselves, although there were some reservations regarding the privacy of their quarters and personal laundry facilities. Heads of Remand Homes showed less satisfaction, and the majority were not fully satisfied regarding privacy and personal cooking facilities. Where an assessment of the accommodation for married staff was given it was generally very favourable, but heads showed considerable dissatisfaction with the accommodation provided for their single staff; this is in contrast to most groups of residential Homes. This was particularly true of the heads of Remand Homes and least marked from heads of Special Schools.

xvi. Remand Homes are generally better placed for shops, cinemas and public transport than either of the other two groups, but two-thirds of all schools and homes are within 20 minutes walk of shops.

xvii. 56 per cent of the full-time care staff at Approved Schools have some formal qualifications, and at Remand Homes and Special Schools 38 per cent are qualified. Schools for the maladjusted or for the physically handicapped employ a higher proportion of qualified staff than do schools for the educationally sub-normal, the blind or the deaf. The proportion of care staff who have some qualification is higher in these schools and remand Homes than almost any other type of residential establishment covered by our survey, except mother and baby Homes.

1. SIZE OF SCHOOLS

177. Heads were asked to give the total number of children in residence. In the case of Special Schools this included a small proportion (7·5 per cent) who attended daily but did not live in.

178. The average number of children varies considerably with the type of establishment. (See Table 4.45). For both Approved Schools for girls and Remand Homes the average unit is small (approximately 30 children), while the average Approved School for boys is three times the size. Special Schools for maladjusted children are also small, averaging 25 children. Those for the educationally sub-normal and the physically handicapped are more than twice as large on average (62 and 54 respectively) and those for the blind and for the deaf average have four times as many children (104).

2. CHILDREN

(a) *Approved Schools and Remand Homes*

179. The 89 Approved Schools and 54 Remand Homes had, at the time of the survey, 8,188 children—7,206 boys and 982 girls (all resident). The ratio of boys to girls was higher for the approved Schools (7·7 to 1) than for the Remand Homes (6 to 1).

180. Girls at Approved Schools and Remand Homes were fairly evenly divided between two age groups—under 15 and 16 to 20, but two-thirds of the boys at Approved Schools and three-quarters of boys at Remand Homes were in the younger group.

(b) *Special Schools*

181. The 399 Special Schools had 22,238 children (20,583 resident in the school) attending them at the time of the survey. The proportion who were not resident but attended daily varied, of course, with the type of disability for which the School was designed. One in five of those attending schools for the deaf and partially deaf was non-resident, as was one in ten of those attending the large group of schools and homes for the educationally sub-normal. Among the remaining Special Schools the proportion of non-residents was small.

182. There are more boys than girls in Special Schools, not because the incidence of handicap is different for the sexes, but handicapped girls are more often cared for at home. At schools and homes for the

maladjusted, boys outnumber girls by four to one; at the other types of school the ratio was much lower.

Table 4.44
Overall Ratio of Boys to Girls in Special Schools

Schools for: Blind and Partially Blind	Deaf and Partially Deaf	Phys. Handicapped	Educ. Sub-normal	Maladjusted	Other	Total
1·5	1·2	1·5	1·8	4·0	2·2	1·7

183. The great majority, about 90 per cent, of the children resident in these Special Schools were aged between 5 and 15. Only at schools for the physically handicapped—5 per cent—and the educationally sub-normal—1 per cent—was there a small percentage under five years old.

3. RATIO OF CHILDREN TO STAFF

184. The results of converting part-time staff into full-time equivalents and then calculating the ratios of resident children to full-time care staff, are shown in Table 4.45, together with the average number of children in each type of school or home.

Table 4.45
Ratio of Children to each full-time equivalent care staff

	Average number of children	Ratio of children to care staff
Approved Schools for—boys	92	10·3
—girls	32	4·1
Total Approved Schools	76	8·8
Total Remand Homes	27	3·1
Special Schools for—blind or partially blind	105	9·1
—deaf or partially deaf	82	7·9
—physically handicapped	52	4·1
—educationally sub-normal	55	7·9
—maladjusted	25	6·0
—other	105	6·1
Total Special Schools	52	6·1

185. In Approved Schools and Remand Homes the ratio of residents to care staff rises as the average number of residents increases. The ratio is lowest in Remand Homes (3·1 residents to each care staff member) where the average number of residents is only 27. Approved Schools for Girls, with an average size of 32 residents, have a ratio of 4·1 compared with 10·3 in Boys' Approved Schools, which average 92 residents.

186. This very big difference in staffing ratios between boys' approved schools and girls' approved schools is not entirely explained by differences in size. It may in part be due to the fact that the girls do a good deal of the domestic work themselves, and therefore nearly all the staff are care staff. In boys' approved schools, some of the caring functions will be carried out by domestic staff, and therefore not so many care staff are needed. Also, the girls are older on average, and may therefore need more individual attention from staff than groups of younger boys.

187. In Special Schools not only the unit size but also the type of disability naturally affects the number of care staff required. Although schools for the maladjusted are very small on average, their child/staff ratio of 6 to 1 is higher than that of schools for the physically handicapped which have 4·1 residents to each staff member but are of medium size. Schools for the mentally sub-normal are also of medium size but have a resident to staff ratio (7·9) as high as that for the much larger schools for the deaf. Of all the Special Schools, those for the blind and the few unclassified schools average the largest number of residents, and the schools for the blind have the highest child/staff ratio (9·1).

4. CARE STAFF (Q. 8)

188. For the 542 schools and homes covered by the survey, the total number of care staff was 4,891 persons: 798 in approved schools, 3,604 in special schools and 489 in remand Homes. Their composition was as shown in Table 4.46.

189. Each of the three broad categories depends overwhelmingly on full-time care staff. In Special Schools almost two-thirds of the staff is resident in the same building as the children. In both Approved Schools and Remand Homes half the staff is resident in the same building, and a further third of the staff in Approved Schools is resident in separate accommodation. Remand Homes have the highest proportion (two-fifths) of staff completely non-resident.

190. Broad conclusions concerning residence, however, have to be modified when the different types of school are studied separately.

191. Almost three-quarters of the care staff in Approved Schools for

G

girls are resident in the same building, and less than half of the remainder are non-resident. A quarter of the staff in Junior and Intermediate Approved Schools for boys are non-resident, but at those for senior boys few are completely so, the majority living in separate accommodation either in the grounds of the school or outside it. Thus, although of similar average size and high child/staff ratio to the junior schools, the senior Approved Schools have an even smaller proportion of their staff (less than two-fifths) actually resident in the same building as the boys.

Table 4.46
Residence Composition of Care Staff in Schools

	Approved Schools %	Remand Homes %	Special Schools %
Full-time staff:			
Resident in same building	49	48	61
Resident in separate accommodation	32	10	10
Non-resident	11	31	15
	92	89	86
Part-time staff:			
Resident in same building	1	1	2
Resident in separate accommodation	1	—	1
Non-resident	6	10	11
Total	100	100	100

192. Of the Special Schools, those for the physically handicapped have the highest proportion (34 per cent) of non-resident care staff and the lowest proportion (55 per cent) resident in the same building. They are followed by schools for the educationally sub-normal (27 per cent and 63 per cent respectively). These account for two-thirds of the total number of Special Schools. The remaining schools average 14 per cent non-resident, 8 per cent resident in separate accommodation and 78 per cent resident in the same building.

Table 4.47
Residence Composition of Care Staff in Approved Schools,
Remand Homes and Special Schools, by type of school

	Full-time Staff				Part-time Staff		
	Res. same building %	*Res. separate* %	*Non-resident* %	*Total Full-time* %	*Res. same building* %	*Res. separate* %	*Non-resident* %
Approved Schools:							
Boys' Junior and Interm.	44	31	17	92	*	*	8 = 100%
Boys' Senior	37	51	8	96	1	3	—
Girls	72	14	4	90	1	—	9
Total Approved Schools	49	32	11	92	1	1	6
Total Remand Homes	48	10	31	89	1	—	10
Special Schools:							
Blind	75	7	9	91	1	—	8
Deaf	70	7	11	88	2	1	9
Phys. handicapped	53	11	20	84	2	*	14
Educ. subnormal	61	9	16	86	2	1	11
Maladjusted	78	11	4	93	3	—	4
Other	77	4	9	90	—	1	9
Total	61	10	15	86	2	1	11

* less than 0·5 per cent.

5. AGE COMPOSITION OF CARE STAFF (Q. 10)

193. At all the schools and Homes the majority of the care staff is aged from 21 to 49.

Table 4.48
Age Composition of Care Staff in Approved Schools
and Remand Homes

	Approved Schools				
	Boys, Junior and Intermediate %	*Boys, Senior* %	*Girls* %	*Total Approved Schools* %	*Remand Homes* %
Staff Aged:					
Under 21	1	—	1	1	1
21–49	64	74	70	68	69
50 and over	35	26	29	31	30
Total	100	100	100	100	100

194. A third of care staff employed at Junior and Intermediate Approved Schools for boys are aged 50 or more, compared with a quarter of the staff at Approved Schools for senior boys. Very few of the staff at any of these schools are under 21.

195. Special Schools, on the other hand, employ an appreciable number of very young care staff (16 per cent of the overall total) but there are variations by type of school. At schools for the physically handicapped there are as many under 21 (23 per cent) as there are aged 50 and over, while only 4 per cent of the care staff at schools for the maladjusted are under 21. There is less variation in the proportion of older staff employed—approximately a quarter at each type of school except those for the maladjusted, where it is about a fifth.

Table 4.49
Age Composition of Care Staff in Special Schools

Staff Aged	Total	Blind and Partially Blind	Deaf and Partially Deaf	Physically Handicapped	Educationally Subnormal	Maladjusted	Other
	%	%	%	%	%	%	%
Under 21	16	9	17	23	13	4	10
21–49	60	63	56	54	62	75	64
50 and over	24	28	27	23	25	21	26
Total	100	100	100	100	100	100	100

6. SEX AND MARITAL STATUS OF RESIDENT CARE STAFF AND EMPLOYMENT OF THEIR SPOUSES (Q. 11)

196. Of all care staff (full-time and part-time) the majority are resident either in the same accommodation as the children or in separate accommodation in the grounds of the school and outside it (83 per cent of staff at Approved Schools, 59 per cent at Remand Homes and 74 per cent at Special Schools).

197. At the Special Schools, nearly 80 per cent of this resident staff are women and two thirds are single women. At Remand Homes, where there are six times as many boys as girls, two-fifths of the resident staff are women and one-fifth are single women. Although there are eight boys to every girl in Approved Schools, half the resident staff are women because the number of staff in relation to children is much higher in approved schools for girls than it is for boys. The majority of the female care staff resident in Approved Schools are single, but the majority of the male staff are married and a third of the wives work in the school. At Remand Homes nearly two-thirds of the male resident staff are married and more than half the wives also work in the Homes. In the great majority of cases where a married woman is

employed in any of these Homes and schools, her husband is also employed full-time.

Table 4.50
Sex, Marital Status and Employment of Spouses of Resident Care Staff

	Approved Schools %	Remand Homes %	Special Schools %
Married women:			
Husband working full-time in Home	12	17	10
Husband working part-time in Home	*	1	1
With husband not working in Home	1	3	3
Married men:			
Wife working full-time in Home	11	19	9
Wife working part-time in Home	1	1	1
With wife not working in Home	23	15	3
Single women	38	19	66
Single men	14	25	7
Total	100	100	100
Total women	51	40	79
Total men	49	60	21
	100	100	100

* less than 0·5 per cent.

198.   Again, there are substantial variations related to type of school. Almost all of the resident care staff at girls' Approved Schools are single women—90 per cent. Of the resident staff at boys' Junior and Intermediate Approved Schools one-quarter are single men and one-quarter single women. A further two-fifths are married men and the remainder are their wives. Approved Schools for senior boys employ a much higher proportion of married men—over half total staff—and only a fifth of the resident care staff are single men or single women (14 per cent and 7 per cent).

199.   Two-thirds of the resident care staff at the Special Schools are single women. Schools for the blind and for the deaf employ most single women (82 per cent and 76 per cent respectively). Schools for the maladjusted depend much more on married couples where both husband and wife work full-time—40 per cent of the staff.

7. STAFF WASTAGE AND REPLACEMENT

For methods of calculation, see survey of old people's Homes, para. 40 above.

    (a) *Replacements and losses of full-time care staff, excluding the head of Homes* (Q. 13a and Q. 14).

200.   Most Schools and Homes show loss rates very similar to other residential Homes—between a quarter and a third of staff left during the year, but boys' approved schools and special schools for the blind and the deaf have appreciably lower loss rates than average.

201.   In most cases, schools and remand Homes lost a higher proportion of resident staff than non-resident staff. There were more losses than replacements among resident posts, but more replacements than losses among non-resident posts. The excess of losses was most marked among resident staff at Remand Homes.

Table 4.51
Annual Gains and Losses for Full-time Care Staff

| | Resident Staff | | Non-resident Staff | | All Staff | |
	Gains %	Losses %	Gains %	Losses %	Gains %	Losses %
Approved Schools:						
Boys, Junior and Inter.	16	15	17	11	16	15
Boys, Senior	14	19	43	29	17	20
Girls	23	28	38	50	24	29
Total App. Schools	17	20	23	17	18	19
Total Remand Homes	24	40	19	14	22	31
Special Schools:						
Blind or partially blind	18	21	14	14	18	21
Deaf or partially deaf	23	22	15	27	22	22
Physically handicapped	29	32	20	19	27	29
Educ. sub-normal	26	29	24	24	26	28
Maladjusted	23	25	44	19	24	24
Other	29	45	7	—	27	41
Total Special Schools	27	29	21	20	26	28

    (b) *New Appointments of full-time client-care staff* (Q. 13b)

202.   The whole sample reported only 106 appointments to new full-time posts during the preceding twelve months; this was equivalent to a 2·5 per cent expansion in full-time care staff. More than half this growth occurred in Approved Schools and more than a third were non-resident posts. However, it would be rash on one year's figures to conclude that this is an established pattern of growth in the staffing of these schools and homes.

(c) Vacancies (Q. 9)

203. Nevertheless, Approved Schools had a higher ratio of vacancies to filled posts than either Remand Homes or Special Schools. At the time of the survey, vacancies for care staff at Approved Schools were equivalent to 9 per cent of total care staff and those that had been unfilled for six months or more were equal to 6 per cent. The position was particularly serious in Approved Schools for girls, where vacancies were 15 per cent of total staff. This is the highest proportion of vacancies in any category of residential establishment.

Table 4.52
Care Staff Vacancies (as a Percentage of Total Care Staff)

	Total Vacancies %	Vacancies Unfilled 6 months %
Approved Schools:		
Boys, junior and interm.	5	3
Boys, senior	8	5
Girls	15	12
Total Approved Schools	9	6
Total Remand Homes	7	1
Total Special Schools	5	2

(d) Reasons for Leaving (Q. 15)

204. These figures will not be published (see explanation in para. 46 above). They are available for consultation at the N.C.S.S. or the N.I.S.W.T.

(e) Turnover of heads of Homes (Q. 16)

205. Turnover was not as high amongst heads of schools and remand Homes as it was in other residential establishments. More than two-thirds of all schools and remand Homes had had only one head for the past five years or more. Special schools showed a remarkable degree of stability; only a quarter had had more than one head in the previous five years. In most other institutions covered in the survey, 40 per cent or more had had more than one head.

Table 4.53
Turnover of Heads of Schools and Remand Homes

| | No. of Heads in Preceding 5 Years | | | |
| | *1 Head* | *2 Heads* | *3 or more* | *Total* |
	%	%	%	%
Approved Schools	67	29	4	100
Remand Homes	71	25	4	100
Special Schools	74	24	2	100

8. VIEWS ON STAFF ACCOMMODATION (Q. 17)

206.   In the survey of old people's Homes (see para. 50 above) we discuss more fully the replies on accommodation. The majority of heads of schools and Homes were satisfied with the accommodation provided, and we do not show separate tables, although they are available for consultation.

207.   More heads of Remand Homes expressed themselves as being dissatisfied with accommodation than the other groups, and heads of all these establishments were not satisfied with the accommodation provided for single staff. This is very different from the attitude of heads of old people's Homes and children's Homes.

(a) *Accommodation for Heads of Schools and Homes*

208.   The majority of the heads of Approved Schools and Special Schools described their own accommodation as completely satisfactory on every aspect. Among heads of Approved Schools a large minority were less than completely satisfied with the privacy of their quarters and the greatest dissatisfaction emerged on the provision of personal laundry facilities. Heads of Remand Homes showed less satisfaction on almost every point. On privacy, in particular, there was a majority who were not fully satisfied and there was considerable dissatisfaction regarding personal cooking facilities.

(b) *Accommodation for other Staff*

209.   When asked to rate the accommodation for their married staff, it was rare for any amenity to be considered completely satisfactory by less than 70 per cent of the respondents. Heads of Remand Homes, however, again showed considerable dissatisfaction with the personal cooking facilities for married staff.

210.   Heads' assessments of the accommodation provided for single care staff was not favourable. Only in the case of the heating facilities at Approved and Special Schools and laundry facilities at Special

Schools was there a substantial majority who were completely satisfied. Heads of Special Schools showed only a small majority completely satisfied on all other points; for personal cooking facilities, there was considerable dissatisfaction expressed by the heads of all three groups of schools.

211. Heads of Approved Schools were very dissatisfied with the privacy and space available for single staff and were far from completely satisfied with the bathroom, lavatory and laundry facilities. Heads of Remand Homes showed even more dissatisfaction with bathroom and lavatory facilities and, again, were dissatisfied with the space available. Only a third were completely satisfied regarding privacy.

9. OTHER ACCOMMODATION AND AMENITIES FOR STAFF
(a) Staff Sitting Room for Exclusive Staff Use
212. Two-thirds of all schools and Homes have a separate staff sitting room, but this provision is considerably less common among Remand Homes and schools for the maladjusted.

(b) Multi-purpose Staff Sitting Room
213. 39 per cent of Special Schools, 42 per cent of Approved Schools and 47 per cent of Remand Homes reported that they had a staff sitting room which was, however, used for other purposes. The incidence of such rooms is generally higher where provision of an exclusive staff sitting room is lower.

(c) Separate Staff Dining Room
214. Only one in every five Remand Homes has a separate dining room, compared with one in three of the Special Schools and one in two Approved Schools. Of the 92 schools for the maladjusted only one in ten has such a room—and this may be compared with three in every ten schools for the educationally sub-normal and half the schools for the physically handicapped.

(c) Combined Dining Room and Sitting Room
215. Approximately half the Approved Schools and Remand Homes have a combined dining room and sitting room. The proportion is slightly less among Special Schools.

(e) Separate Staff Recreation Room
216. There are very few separate staff recreation rooms. 8 per cent of Approved Schools and Special Schools have one, and 4 per cent of Remand Homes.

(f) Changing Room for Non-resident Staff

217. About a quarter of the Approved Schools have a changing room for non-resident staff. The proportion is slightly higher in the Special Schools (30 per cent) and highest in Remand Homes (40 per cent). There is considerable variation between the types of Special School on this point—of the three larger groups, the schools for the physically handicapped are the most likely to have this accommodation (41 per cent), among schools for the educationally sub-normal it is less frequent (28 per cent), and among schools for the maladjusted it is infrequent (15 per cent).

(g) Proximity to Shops, Cinemas, etc.

218. Remand Homes are generally better placed for shopping and recreational facilities than are Approved Schools or Special Schools. 85 per cent of Remand Homes are located within a 20 minute walk of shops, compared with 65 per cent of Approved Schools and 71 per cent of Special Schools. 66 per cent of Remand Homes are within a 20 minute walk of cinemas, dance halls, etc., compared with 50 per cent of Approved Schools and 43 per cent of Special Schools.

(h) Proximity to Public Transport

219. Here again, Remand Homes tend to be less isolated than the other two groups—the great majority (84 per cent) are on a bus route with services at least every half-hour but little more than half the Approved Schools and Special Schools (57 per cent) have as frequent a service to cinemas etc. and only slightly more have one to shops. (61 per cent of Approved Schools and 60 per cent of Special Schools). This means that schools tend to be more isolated than most other types of residential establishments.

10. QUALIFICATIONS[1] OF CARE STAFF

(a) Full-time Staff

220. A comparatively high proportion of staff in Approved Schools are qualified. More than half the full-time care staff at Approved Schools have some formal qualification, but at Remand Homes and Special Schools the proportion of qualified staff is considerably lower (38 per cent).

221. In Approved Schools and Remand Homes, most of the staff who have some recognized qualification have some kind of teaching credential, even though they are not teachers (28 per cent of all care staff in Approved Schools, 18 per cent in Remand Homes). Special Schools for the maladjusted also have a high proportion—19 per cent.

---

* A full list of qualifications is set out in Appendix B.

Table 4.54
Employment of Qualified Full-time Staff

| | Approved Schools | | | | Remand Homes | Special Schools | | | | | | Total |
	Boys, Junior and Inter.	Boys, Senior	Girls	Total		Blind	Deaf	Phys. Hand.	ESN	Mal-adj.	Other	
	%	%	%	%	%	%	%	%	%	%	%	%
Nursing qualifs.	4	3	9	5	6	9	9	19	9	6	22	13
Cert. Resid. Child Care or equiv.	19	6	18	16	8	9	8	8	12	15	1	9
N.N.E.B., etc.	*	—	—	*	*	1	2	3	1	2	—	2
Cert. of Educ.	24	17	11	18	13	7	5	5	12	15	1	8
Craft teachg.	7	21	7	10	5	3	4	1	4	4	1	3
Dom. Science	1	4	9	4	1	2	6	2	3	4	1	3
Univ. Degree	6	8	4	6	4	2	5	1	2	4	3	2
Soc. Sci. Dip.	2	2	5	3	1	1	—	*	1	6	—	1
Other	1	1	4	2	*	1	1	2	2	1	2	2
None	43	46	44	44	62	65	66	59	65	56	80	62
Total**	107	108	111	108	100	100	106	100	111	113	111	105

* less than 0·5 per cent.
** More than 100 per cent because some staff have more than one qualification.

In Special Schools as a whole, only 11 per cent have teaching qualifications and 13 per cent have nursing qualifications. Staff with nursing qualifications are, as expected, found mainly in schools for the physically handicapped, and in the 'other schools'.

222. In Approved Schools and in schools for the maladjusted and E.S.N. quite a high proportion have taken residential child care training (16, 15 and 12 per cent respectively). This is particularly marked in girls' and in junior boys' Approved Schools.

(b) Part-time Staff

223. Of the comparatively small numbers of part-time care staff employed, a third of those in Approved Schools are qualified, but less than a fifth of those in Special Schools and very few (6 per cent) of those in Remand Homes.

5

THE FUTURE DEMAND

1. We come now to the most hazardous part of our Report—an attempt to estimate the future demand for residential care; hazardous because it depends on so many factors each of which is capable of variation within wide limits. We first set out these factors briefly so that it may be clear how inevitably speculative our estimates are.

2. ## I. DEMOGRAPHIC TRENDS

(a) The number of old people (whenever we use this phrase we refer to those over 65) can be known with reasonable precision. Those who have a chance of reaching the age of 65 within the next sixty years have already been born and, unless death rates at different ages undergo a remarkable change, we can calculate how many men and women will be classed as 'old' for each year to come. But, as we have seen, the proportion of those in the early part of old age who need residential care is nothing like so large as that of the very old. (According to our own figures, 49 per cent of those in residential Homes are over 80). It follows then that the number of old people for whom provision must be made depends on the expectation of life amongst the really aged, and this has changed and may change even more dramatically with improvements in medical knowledge.

3. The number of the old who need care—from sources other than their own families—is influenced, again, by the marriage rates. On the whole few married people come into care. In 1958–9, for example, only 0.25 per cent of married people over 65 were in Homes, whilst the proportion was 8 per cent of single men, 4 per cent of widowers, 4 per cent of single women and 1 per cent of widows. If we take instead the later age of 75 and over, we find the same differences:

·7 per cent of married people, 12 per cent of single men, 6 per cent of widowers, 8 per cent of single women and 3 per cent of widows.[1]

4. The marriage rates current in the decades when the present old people were young were very much lower than they are today. Of the women born in the first decade of this century, about 15 per cent remained permanently unmarried; today, only about 5 per cent of young women are single. There seems a probability, then, that a smaller proportion of this larger number of the elderly will need care in the more distant future because a larger proportion of them will be married, but this will not become effective until the end of this century.

5. When we come to other groups, however, we have much less firm ground on which to stand.

(b) Birth rates and family sizes constantly change and these changes are unpredictable. Since 1942 the birth rate has shown great vagaries. Before that year there was a consistent downward trend to the all-time low of 14·4 per thousand of the population in 1941; since then we have first had the big upward surge until 1947 ('the bulge') but although the rate fell from the high peak of that year it has not since demonstrated any definite trend. Some years it has risen, some it has fallen, though never to the low level of the thirties. During most of the fifties it ranged between 15 and 16 but it has risen during the sixties. The latest figure, that for 1965, is 18·3. We cannot, therefore, say with any degree of certainty how many children of different ages there are likely to be at future dates. Yet the more children there are—or the fewer—the more or less are at risk in needing care.

6. (c) It is even less possible to predict what proportion of the children born will be handicapped physically or mentally and we are even more in the dark in guessing how many may become emotionally disturbed because of the circumstances of their lives.

7. (d) The growth of medical knowledge helps to reduce the numbers of severely handicapped children but it also continually increases the number of the handicapped who remain alive. This adds a further unknown to our calculations of those likely to need care.

---

[1] W. Beckerman and Associates, *The British Economy in 1975*, Cambridge University Press, Table 13.11.

II. SOCIAL POLICY

8. The proportion of those needing residential care varies according to the social policies of the time.

 (a) A marked increase in the rates of pensions for old people and widows or of family allowances, might make it possible for more old people and children to remain in their own homes.

9. (b) A significant development in domiciliary services or the provision of more sheltered housing would also reduce the number of those seeking admission to Homes: for example, more home helps and visiting nurses, or the regular provision of more hot nourishing meals, would enable many to continue living at home up to a much greater age than at present, and might make it possible for more children to remain at home during a temporary crisis. Those who live in sheltered housing with a warden and the provision of some communal services usually do not need to move into residential Homes. The further development of Day Care facilities for all kinds of handicapped and infirm people would allow of a reduction in the number of residential Homes required because all those using these Day Centres return to their families for the night.

10. It should be understood that we are not at this point expressing any view with regard to the desirability or otherwise of such services; we are merely pointing out that the extent to which they are provided necessarily influences the number of those for whom residential establishments must be provided. How wide the variations may be, due to these and similar factors, can be seen from the present figures. The Ministry of Health has published statements compiled from the returns of local authorities of England and Wales, showing the provision for old people that they intend to make ten years ahead. Although the Ministry gives some general guidance, a great deal is left to local discretion and in the latest Ten Year Plan published, the number of residential places in existence for old people varied from 6 per thousand of the population over 65 in the locality to 32. There are, of course, many reasons for such wide divergencies—the age structure of the population and the socio-economic conditions—but something must be due to the differences in the alternative provisions available. If all authorities moved in either direction to an extreme degree any estimate made on present circumstances would be derisory.

11. (c) There is considerable division of opinion as to where very old and frail persons can be best cared for. Professor

Townsend has even argued that there may be no need for old people's Homes at all if, on the one hand, there were adequate domiciliary services and sheltered housing and, on the other, good geriatric wards in hospitals. Others maintain that it is unkind to move old people from their familiar environment when they are least able to adjust themselves. Whatever may be the merits or demerits of these arguments we are concerned here to show how largely our estimates of needs must depend on social policies which we cannot predict.

III. SOCIAL AND ECONOMIC CHANGES

12. One of the outstanding characteristics of contemporary life is the increase in personal mobility. There have, of course, been many periods during the last two hundred years when large numbers of people have moved from their old homes because of profound economic changes; the movement from the country to the towns throughout much of the last century, for example, and the exodus from the mining and shipbuilding areas during the twenties and early thirties of this century. But there are now many more factors in operation which combine to make movement a constant, rather than an exceptional, feature of life. Population statistics show that the midlands and the south-eastern areas of the country have added to the number of their inhabitants by very much more than the national average whilst the north-east and much of Wales show exactly the opposite. And inside all these areas there is a constant change in relative densities.

13. Part of this is the result of improvements in communications. It is no longer essential to live close to one's work and hundreds of thousands of workers leave the congested centres of towns and make their homes twenty or thirty miles from their work. Part of this movement is also due to deliberate policy. Local authority housing estates and other new residential suburbs are sited away from the industrial and commercial centres so as to get the advantage of lower ground rents and a healthier environment. In the attempt to prevent the increasing congestion in the large conurbations, New Towns, complete with industry, commerce, schools and all the necessary amenities of life are planned and established in what were rural areas or small country towns; and many inducements are offered to encourage both employers and workers to move to them.

14. When people do move, whether it is to take advantage of better housing or a more attractive and healthy neighbourhood or because of the better opportunities for employment, they do not usually take the

older generation with them[1] and it would only be by coincidence that their brothers and sisters, with their families, moved at the same time and to the same place. This means that in times of stress a family is likely to be stranded without the assistance of their kinsfolk simply because they have no relatives in the same neighbourhood. A woman who is ill or about to have a new baby has no mother or sister living in the next street who can take care of the children whilst she is in hospital; and the old folks who remain in the old neighbourhood have nobody to help with the shopping and washing.

15. Even when families live close to one another it is more difficult to accommodate those in need than it used to be because of the higher standards of living which are now the acceptable minimum. When houses and their equipment were on a much lower scale than now, a good deal of discomfort was taken for granted because of the lack of any alternative. An extra person or two could be squeezed in by improvising beds on the kitchen sofa or by crowding another person into the children's bedroom. This is no longer acceptable. Many old people, however devoted they may be to their children and grand-children, do not want to live with them; and younger prople who have become accustomed to the higher standards of today would not tolerate the degree of overcrowding that their parents were forced to accept in less affluent times. Such constantly changing ideas of what is acceptable have an important effect on the number of those for whom the ordinary family provision cannot be made.

IV. THE IMPONDERABLES

16. (a) It is sometimes thought that a decline in family affection is a major contributory cause of the increase in the number of those in need of care. There is no evidence for such a statement. Indeed what evidence we have leads in the opposite direction. The various studies made in recent years show how strong kinship ties still are and the great efforts made by the majority of people to care for those directly related to them. Where family cohesion has lessened it has mainly been because of the factors mentioned in the preceding paragraphs.

17. Yet at the same time it must be accepted that the modern concept of 'the family' is very different from that of our grandfathers. While we still, no doubt, feel great affection for 'our sisters and our cousins and

[1] There is some evidence however that people tend to join their children in advanced old age.

our aunts' we do not today feel ourselves so strongly bound to them or so intimately involved in their fortunes as used to be customary a hundred years ago. It is, therefore, possible that further changes may take place. As things are now, we look after those of our family who are old or disabled or in distress, not only because of natural affection, but because there are strong social pressures which mould our ideas of what is the right course of action. We make efforts to match up to what is expected of us because we fear the criticism of our friends or neighbours or because we are afraid of the nagging of our own consciences. But if the general ideas of what constitutes family obligations underwent further radical changes our behaviour would change too; and this would have a great effect on the demand for communally provided residential care.

18.   (b) There is little doubt that, at present, living in a 'Home' however charming and well run, is considered a second best to normal family life by the majority of people; but we are not sure that this attitude will necessarily persist. Many people of considerable means nowadays voluntarily give up their own homes and live in hotels or other ways of group living at the seaside or in pleasant country towns. This development began on a large scale soon after the war when food shortages and the lack of domestic help put unfamiliar burdens on many households that were geared to a different way of living; but it has persisted and grown because so many people have found it agreeable. Looking at TV is more enjoyable when one can discuss the programme with others; a game of cards is possible without the need to invite others in for the purpose and there are all sorts of additions to social life that help one to pass the time agreeably. The purpose-built Homes for old people now being built are usually delightfully planned and well equipped; if they further develop to give their residents help in living an interesting and sociable life it could easily happen that a much larger proportion than at present would choose to live in them rather than maintain their separate homes. It is significant that the proportion of the elderly living in Homes is very much lower in this country than in many others. It was estimated that in 1963 there were 105,000 old people, i.e. 1·7 per cent of the population aged 65 and over living in Homes, including both local authority and voluntary Homes.[1] In Holland, on

---

[1] *The Aged in the Welfare State*, Townsend & Wedderburn. Occasional Papers on Social Administration, No. 14.

the other hand, a much higher proportion of those over 65 live in old people's Homes.

ESTIMATES OF FUTURE NEEDS

19. For all these reasons we do not feel ourselves able to make any definite estimate of future needs. Yet *some* estimate we must make if our recommendations are to be of any value. We are proposing certain very radical changes and, in particular, are recommending the establishment of courses of training, and there would be no point in doing so unless we could reach some tentative conclusions about the size of the problem to be faced.

20. In view of these many variable factors, therefore, we decided to limit ourselves in two ways:

(i) We made the calculations on which we venture only for the next ten years or so. On the whole, changes in patterns of living and in social ideas do not alter in a revolutionary way in a short period and the variables are, thus, likely to be less indefinite in so short a period as 10 or 15 years. Yet at the same time it is a long enough period to give some indication of trends.

21. (ii) We make our estimates for only two groups—the old people's Homes and children's Homes. We have chosen these partly because they are by far the most numerous of all those with whom we are concerned and partly because we have more established facts to guide us.

OLD PEOPLE IN RESIDENTIAL HOMES

22. How many old people will there be? And how many of these are likely to require residential care? According to the population projections made by the Registrar-General the number of men and women over 65 in 1980 will have risen from the present total of 6,560,000 to 8,210,000—an increase of nearly a million and three quarters—of whom nearly two-thirds will be women. But as we have seen, the clientele at present in residential homes is heavily weighted in the older age groups so it is necessary to consider what proportion of this total of old people will fall into different ages.

This means that 5 per cent of the total population will be over 75 and 2·3 per cent over 80, the groups which form the biggest groups now in Homes.

23. What proportion of these numbers is likely to require residential care, taking into account as far as possible the factors to which reference

Table 5.1

*Total U.K. Population and Population in the Older Age Groups,
1965 and 1980 (millions)**

| | 1965 | | | 1980 | | |
	Men	Women	Total	Men	Women	Total
Total population	26·60	28·00	54·60	30·12	31·11	61·22
Total population 65+	2·49	4·07	6·56	3·25	4·96	8·21
Total population 75+	·79	1·57	2·36	1·01	2·01	3·02
Total population 80+	·35	·76	1·11	·40	·99	1·39

* Annual Abstract of Statistics, 1966, Table 12.

was made earlier? For this we have some help from a study made by the
National Institute for Economic and Social Research,[1] which has made
an estimate of the likely demand for residential care in the health and
welfare services in 1975, and by several other studies of those in Homes
made by Professor Townsend.[2] A sample survey made by Townsend
and Wedderburn for the year 1962-3 shows the great difference in the
proportions of the population in institutions according to family
status.

Table 5.2

Marital and Family Status of persons aged 65 and over[3]

| | In Institutions | | | In Private Households | | |
| | Men | Women | Men and Women | Men | Women | Men and Women |
	%	%	%	%	%	%
Unmarried	32	34	33	4	14	10
Married or widowed but childless	24	28	26	16	16	16

24.   How does this affect the probabilities for the next ten or fifteen
years? Not very much so far as the first line of figures in Table 5.2 is
concerned. Those who will reach the ages of 70 to 80 by 1980 will have
been born in the early years of this century and of these a large proportion of women remained unmarried. This was due partly to the
fact that the mortality rates for boys was much higher than that for
girls so that there were more marriageable women than men; and

[1] Wilfred Beckermann and Associates *The British Economy in 1975*, Cambridge
University Press 1965. Chapter VI by K. Jones and D. Paige.
[2] P. Townsend *The Last Refuge*, and Townsend and Wedderburn *The Aged in the
Welfare State*.
[3] Op. cit., Townsend and Wedderburn.

partly to the very high death rate of young men during the first World War. It is only since the second World War that both these factors have undergone a revolutionary change. Nowadays the number of men in the marriage ages exceeds that of young women and there has been a consequent dramatic increase in the proportion of women marrying; but the effect of this will not be seen on the marital status of the old for 30 or 40 years.

25. But when we come to the second line of figures in the table it is a different matter. The decrease in the birth rate and the increase in the proportion of childless families and of families with only two or three children had already begun to be significant by the time that those born in the early years of the century reached the age to marry. The birth rate reached its lowest point in the late thirties and those who were married in the twenties and thirties generally had small families. In 1960 18·5 per cent of married or widowed old people had no surviving child, 18 per cent had only one surviving child and 43 per cent had three or more. It is estimated that by 1975 22 per cent will have no surviving child, 24·5 per cent will have one and only 30 per cent will have three or more.[1]

26. If past circumstances, then, are any guide to the future we must expect that a large proportion of the elderly will want residential accommodation simply on account of the lack of any close family to care for them. How much this may be still further increased by the factors we have listed as Social and Economic Factors and by the Imponderables it is impossible to guess. Yet we believe that the effect will be to increase the proportion to a considerable extent. The present generation of elderly lived their early years in the shadow of the work-house and the many old people who now refuse to ask for the supplementary allowances to retirement pensions to which they have a right is evidence of the power this experience still has to condition their thinking. The new type of Home for the old has become more usual only since 1948 and there are, unhappily, still a very large number of the old buildings in use (though the treatment of those who live in them has altered so greatly). But in another ten or fifteen years fewer old people will have memories of the 'bad old days' and more will have become familiar with the pleasant conditions now provided. It is likely that this, as well as the effect of rising expectations in private homes with their corollary of the difficulty of fitting in extra people, will make for an increase in the numbers wishing for residential care.

27. There is one factor which might work in the contrary direction. Retirement pensions are almost certain to rise—the rise in the numbers

[1] Op. cit. Beckermann and others, p. 432.

of old people who are voters makes this a fairly certain political prophecy!—and there is a strong movement towards the provision of more services such as sheltered housing and various domiciliary services, which enable people to remain longer in their own homes. But it is impossible to calculate to what extent this might counteract the other trends.

28.   The estimate by the N.I.E.S.R. to which reference was made earlier, envisages a substantial increase in the numbers of places required for old people. According to their calculations, by 1975 2·4 per cent of the population of old people will need places in Homes, even if one million new sheltered houses have been built. This would mean an increase to 165,000 places in England and Wales, or an addition of 68,000 over 1960.

Table 5.3
Numbers aged 65 and over in Old People's Homes 1960 and 1975[1]

	1960		1975	
		percentage of population over 65		*percentage of population over 65*
Welfare Homes L.A.	64,500	1·2		
Sponsored places[2]	9,400	·2	138,000	2·0
Voluntary and Private Homes	22,800	·4	27,000	·4
Total	96,700	1·8	165,000	2·4

29.   This estimate is confirmed by the Local Authorities' Ten Year Plan. By 1976 the local authorities in England and Wales expect to need places for 2·2 per cent of old people, which means that 147,000 places will be needed (excluding 7,000 persons under 65 living in Homes for the elderly). If we add to this figure those who are likely to be accommodated in Homes provided by voluntary organizations, the estimate of 165,000 does not seem extravagant. This means that compared with an estimated 130,000 old people in residential care today[3],

---

[1] Op. cit. Beckerman and Associates, Table 13.12.

[2] Accommodation provided for Local Authorities by voluntary organizations.

Estimate based on the number of places in local authority Homes for the elderly but excluding those under 65, plus the number of residents in voluntary and other Homes registered under the National Assistance Act including those in Homes for the old and disabled, 31st December, 1965. (Annual Report of the Ministry of Health, 1965 Cmnd. 3039.)

we must anticipate an increase of 27 per cent in the demand; i.e. for every 10 old people who were in residential care in 1965, there may be 13 in 1975.

30. In Scotland a comparable rate of increase is envisaged. There were at the end of 1965, 7,489 old people in local authority Homes in Scotland and 5,400 in voluntary homes. It is anticipated that provision will need to be made for some 15,740 altogether by 1971, a 22 per cent increase in six years.

31. What does this figure of 165,000 places in England and Wales alone mean for staffing? If staffing ratios remain as they are at present, i.e. an average of 6·3 residents to each member of staff[1] 5,400 more staff would be needed (apart from replacement of wastage) by 1975. But we give reasons in our later chapters for the view that this ratio is too low. The larger proportions of infirm and mentally disturbed old people, due to the preponderance of the very old, the overwork of staffs, and the lack of adequate free time and holidays, all point to the importance of increasing the staffs of Homes for old people. The N.I.E.S.R. estimate decided that a ratio of 4·3:1 would be required. Such a formidable increase would require almost double the numbers employed today! If we took a more conservative estimate, say, half way between that and the present ratio, we get an increase of 50 per cent, or over 10,000 more staff in ten years' time.

Table 5.4
Estimates of staff required with different ratios of residents to care staff

	1965	1975		
Residents	130,000	165,000	165,000	165,000
Ratio of Residents to Staff	6·3	6·3	5·3	4·3
Staff required	20,600	26,000	31,000	38,000

CHILDREN IN RESIDENTIAL CARE

32. We have given reasons for the great difficulty in making any estimate of the numbers of children likely to need residential care. We cannot know how many children will have been born in the late seventies, for this depends on birth rates which are much less steady in trend than they used to be. If rates remain more or less the same as now, there will be about 17,500,000 children under 18 by the mid-seventies compared with 15,200,000 in 1965. If the same proportions

[1] Staff ratio figures given in Chapter IV, Table 4.8.

were to be in residential care this would involve 5,000 new places. If the staff ratios in children's Homes remained the same, it would mean 1,300 extra staff in children's Homes.

33. But will even the proportion of children in Homes remain the same? We don't know. Social work on behalf of children has undergone considerable changes and is likely to continue to do so. For example, since 1963 local authorities have had a statutory responsibility to give guidance and assistance to families in need with a view, where possible, to preserving the family as a unit. The results of this work in terms of the number of children coming into residential care cannot be measured accurately. It is impossible to estimate even in general terms the future demand that there is likely to be unless there is an accepted policy about which children should receive residential care. The definition of the need changes as society itself changes. As wealth and psychological knowledge increase we become more sophisticated in our standards of what is acceptable. It is probable that increased affluence reduces the demand due to poverty; but on the other hand, not only might higher standards of child care be demanded but there might be an increased number of children with emotional problems who need help in a residential setting.

34. Again one of the factors which determines the number of children who need residential care is the policy and success of the local authority in boarding children out with foster parents. Some authorities foster nearly all the children for whom they are responsible; others only about a third. It may be that those in the latter category would foster more if they could find suitable people; it may be, however, that the proportion of children than can be fostered has reached a plateau. There are differing views on this and some of our witnesses suggested that, with the rising proportion of children coming into care because of emotional disturbances, fewer can be successfully placed in foster homes. It is evident, therefore, that there are similar imponderables to be taken into account as in the case of old people and this makes any attempt at an estimate little more than a guess. The only firm fact on which we can plan is that the numbers of children in the population as a whole is increasing and that there is, at least, a strong possibility that a larger number, though not necessarily a larger proportion, will need residential care.

35. We said earlier that we would confine even these halting estimates to the two groups of the old and children because we have so little information of any others. A word or two can, however, be said about them. As far as approved schools are concerned we can make no estimate at all, for their future depends on the action decided as a result

of current deliberations—in England and Wales and in Scotland—about the future organization of social work. Similarly we can make no guess of the number of places that might be needed in mother and baby Homes. There is nothing precise that can be said of the future of boarding special schools; insofar as possible, handicapped children are educated in non-residential schools, and although some extra provision of boarding places is anticipated, the increase is not expected to be very large.

36. On the other hand, the numbers and places for such groups as the physically and mentally handicapped which figure in the Ten Year Plan of the Local Authorities are expected to show a considerable increase. Indeed there are certain of these which show a dramatic increase—that is, hostels for the mentally ill and the mentally sub-normal, are expected to increase at least five-fold, as is shown by the following table.

Table 5.5

	1965	1976
L.A. Hostels for the mentally sub-normal		
Premises	122	545
No. of Residents	2,346	11,560
L.A. Hostels for the mentally ill		
Premises	41	259
No. of Residents	813	4,966

The implication of these figures for staffing requirements need hardly be stressed.

37. Though our estimates are necessarily inadequate in accuracy, there can be little doubt that there will be a very considerable increase in the numbers required for staffing residential Homes during the next ten or fifteen years. In a later chapter we discuss the ways in which these may be recruited and the sources from which they might be drawn. Here we wish only to emphasize certain factors that are of such importance that it is essential to draw attention constantly to them. These relate to the remarkable changes that have taken place in the structure of the population. Three times as many young women marry before they reach the age of 20 as they did at the end of the last century and hardly any women remain unmarried. This is the revolutionary change which is not yet fully recognized but which must now be taken into account in any question which relates to the deployment of the man and woman power of the community. Nearly all women marry, most marry young and the majority have their children during the first

5 to 8 years of their married lives. Young women are no longer an important part of the labour force. Practically all girls enter paid employment between school and marriage but with a rising school age and a lowered age of marriage this period gets shorter and shorter, so young women are a fast disappearing section of the working population. Every occupation which has depended on them in the past must now reconsider its situation.

38.   When we remember that two-thirds of the people at present employed in residential Homes are single women and one-third of all staff are over 50 years of age and, therefore, likely to retire within the next ten years, we can realize how serious this is for residential Homes. In Chapter VII we discuss some of the ways in which this challenge may be met.

6

CONDITIONS OF WORK

1. Residential work has special strains. This is a fact that must always be kept in mind. Care has to be provided for twenty-four hours a day, seven days a week and this means that the pattern of the working week which has become so common in most types of modern work—the five-day week and the short working day—are more difficult to arrange for those who are taking care of people in residence. Not only is the work generally physically exacting and emotionally exhausting but those who undertake it often feel cut off from the activities of the community outside their doors, as well as from their own family and friends and their professional colleagues.

2. Stress has already been laid on the changed character of those in care. For the most part people live in Homes because of some special difficulty. This varies widely from maladjustment or delinquency, to illegitimate pregnancies, homelessness, physical handicap, or mental subnormality or the failing finances and frailty of old age. Whatever may be the causes that make it difficult for them to remain in an ordinary family circle, these are not circumstances that predispose to a tranquil mind.

3. Nevertheless, we have been impressed on our visits to every kind of institution, as well as by the statements of witnesses who came to speak to us, by the large number of people who find happiness in this work, and by the number who declared that they would be unwilling to change it for any other job. It may be that there is a difference in this respect between the satisfactions felt by heads of Homes and those in assistant positions. It is significant that our Census shows that whilst 60 per cent of heads had remained in their jobs for over five years, an average of one in four of assistant staff leave every year. This high rate of turnover amongst those who are, on the whole, the younger members of staffs, cannot be ignored. The long hours of duty (for even if there is little actual work to be done they must remain 'on call') and, more important, the need to undertake evening and week-end duties when

their contemporaries are at leisure, are said to comprise one of the chief factors causing younger staff to leave. Time off when their friends are at work does not compensate adequately for their exclusion from the normal leisure time activities of their age group. 'They are all right until they get a steady boy friend', said one matron; 'then they are off'. And no doubt there are some who are afraid that they never *will* acquire the boy-friend if they are working when most other people are playing.

4.   But whilst this is obviously a special problem for the younger members of staff it is a difficulty for all, whatever their age and status. 'Residential work needs men and women who are tremendously alive, brimming over with mental and spiritual vitality,' said one tutor to us. This is impossible unless they have time and freedom to form and develop their own personal relationships outside the Home and for this they need assured periods of leisure and personal liberty and privacy.

5.   There are, of course, emergencies which must take precedence of any individual claim. This is true in normal family circumstances just as much as in communal Homes. But short of such crises, the members of staff should know some time ahead, and with certainty, when and for how long they are free of duty. It is frustrating to make plans, whatever they may be—to visit friends, to do one's shopping, to join a class or club of one's own interest—if one can never be sure that one will be able to carry them out.

6.   What hours do people actually work? It is impossible to make any valid generalizations. As far as children's Homes are concerned we have some evidence from the daily diaries of housemothers and assistant housemothers in Local Authority Children's Homes quoted from the Social Survey Report in 1960–61, and from the answers to a questionnaire carried out by the Association of Hospital and Welfare Administrators (Children's Homes) over a number of recent years. The first showed a working day of $13\frac{1}{2}$ hours, which included time spent on meals taken with the children but excluded two hours off duty during the day. On a basis of a $5\frac{1}{2}$ day week this gives a working week of 75 hours and it is, perhaps, not surprising that 50 per cent of the housemothers who left said that hours were longer than they had anticipated. In the second case, 85 per cent of heads of Homes said that their hours of duty were 60–70 a week and 100 per cent said they were on call day and night.

7.   For other types of residential Homes there is no comparable evidence and it may be that work with children inevitably involves longer hours on duty than other forms of care. Yet we got the impression that, in very many cases, whatever the age or type of resident for

whom the Home cared, the senior staff were on duty, even if not actually at work, for very long hours. Several employing bodies told us, in fact, that although shorter hours were accepted in principle, the staffing position was so grave that it was in practice impossible for the staff to enjoy such privileges as, for example, a five-day week.

8. Since the war, there has been a marked tendency for the working week to be shortened in most occupations, and it is understandable that the long hours of residential workers should be disliked, particularly when these hours must include evenings and week-ends when others are enjoying leisure. There are certainly many who have been employed in this work for years who philosophically accept the necessity that their working week does not fit into the accepted contemporary pattern, but there is little doubt that this deters some younger people from offering themselves when there are so many alternative occupations which provide an outlet for the same eagerness to do a worth-while job, but without the need to cut oneself off from the companionship of friends and relatives.

9. How to reconcile the needs of the Home with those of the staff is not easy to determine. To say that hours should be short enough to enable the staff to take a part in normal life does not take one very far. In some fields of residential care, the hours of assistant staff are already fixed at 40 a week, plus a reasonable amount of overtime when necessary. This practice should be extended, together with provision for a definite period of free time each day, a day and a half free each week (as a minimum), and a long week-end every month. But for senior staff—heads of Homes or others with special responsibility—the problem is more difficult. Many heads of Homes have told us that they would dislike a fixed working week as they are too conscious of the responsibility they carry and would resent any implication that theirs is a 9–5 job. We would hesitate to make any proposal which might lead the senior staff to feel that we underestimate this heavy responsibility; and, indeed, at a time when people in this work wish to establish themselves in the public mind as a profession with professional standards of behaviour, it would be unwise to lay down too rigorous a pattern. In any crisis or emergency the responsible officer must, of course, respond over and above the hours of duty laid down whatever they may be. Nevertheless, it is fortunate that crises do not occur every day, and much can be done if employing bodies make provision which allows a reasonable norm of leisure, even though it is well understood that this must be sacrificed when circumstances demand. This depends primarily on the number of people employed and the skill with which the rotas of duty are organized.

10.   Many establishments already consider a 40 hour week suitable for senior staff though many others have not introduced this. We believe that this norm should be more widely applied and that the maximum set as a norm should never be more than 45 hours a week. In some Homes, particularly those providing for children, it is difficult to lay down any hard and fast rules, for in order to create a sense of a real home life, the staff share the meals and recreation of the children. But it is important that employing authorities should recognize the inroads on the private life of the staff that this and other necessities of the job entail and take this fully into account in other aspects of the conditions of employment. Where, for example, long hours on duty are inevitable, it should be possible to make some compensation by longer periods of completely free time and by longer holidays.

11.   At present there is wide variation in practice, from those organizations which give one free day a week and an occasional week-end off, to the few who provide two free days a week, and a long week-end every month in addition to annual leave. In some cases one long day on duty alternates with one free day (and many staff prefer this); in others there are four long working days followed by three free ones. There are so many possible variations and it is so important that flexibility should be preserved that we should not dream of proposing any definite schedule. But whatever the system decided upon there are certain matters that should be kept in mind. First and foremost it is essential that the free times should be definite and arranged sufficiently far ahead for people to make plans which they know they will be able to carry out. Free time is little real benefit if it is haphazard and, although the large majority of people in this kind of work are ready to give up their own pleasures when an emergency arises, care should be taken that the cry of 'Wolf' is not heard too often and only when the gleam of its eyes is already visible.

12.   Again it must be remembered that in order to have a complete rest and change members of staff must have the freedom to spend their free time as they like. One of the most enjoyable ways of using a free day is to potter around at home and do all the odd jobs for which there are not time and energy on a working day. Only too often this is impossible because there is nowhere for an off time to be spent away from the working atmosphere. It is often difficult, particularly in children's Homes, to find a place away from the noise and bustle and few people have a home of their own near enough for a visit. If all off duty days and every week-end off must be spent away from the Home if rest is to be enjoyed, fares and hotel bills soon become overwhelming.

13. A number of devices have been tried by some employers and more experiment in this field is needed. A bungalow or flat which could be booked in advance might prove useful, provided always there was no compulsion on members of staff to use it if they did not wish; or such provision might be made available for all the Homes in an area so that there might be an opportunity of meeting other people in one's time off. (Yet it is only right to add that when we visited one establishment where such provision is made, not one member of staff mentioned its existence to us). As an alternative, more employing bodies might be prepared to pay fares, say, in excess of 10s, two or three times a year or give staff an adequate subsistence allowance on their time off. Such assistance should not, in our view, be considered a substitute for good pay and conditions, but it might be offered as a fringe benefit to offset some of the disadvantages of the awkward hours of duty necessitated by the job.

14. In many Homes four weeks annual leave plus bank holidays (or time off in lieu) is provided but we have met a good many heads who were unable to take their leave because of the lack of a responsible deputy to take charge. In such exacting work it is essential for there to be a real break and the more responsible the job the greater is the need. Some people prefer a number of short holidays to one long one and there is room for many variations on a general pattern but what is important is the recognition that the nature of the work is such that special care must be taken to ensure that the staff have some adequate break from work whatever the form it takes. A good case can be made out, for example, for the offer of sabbatical leave for those carrying heavy responsibility. If heads of Homes could look forward to six or eight weeks extra leave after, say, ten years of service, there might be real encouragement to remain in the work. We realize that there are problems attached to such a provision; for the relief staff would almost of necessity have to occupy the accommodation during the regular staff's absence and this is not always welcomed. But, after all, this has long been accepted as part of the pattern of existence in overseas jobs, whether those in Government or industrial service and has not led to serious difficulties. This is quite different from the use of staff accommodation during normal weekly free times off when extra accommodation should be provided as part of the ordinary equipment of the Home. (In the questionnaire prepared by the Association of Hospital and Welfare Administrators (Children's Section) for instance, one-third of the staff said they had to vacate their room whenever they went away so that the relief staff could use them. This meant that they could never think of their rooms as their homes, but only as lodgings.)

15. The provision of adequate free time depends primarily on the number of staff employed. Some Homes are seriously understaffed, not only on account of the difficulty in recruiting suitable people, but because the employing body has unrealistic ideas of what can reasonably be expected. We have visited old people's Homes where the Matron was the only member of staff on the premises after 3 p.m. every day. One mother and baby Home for 12 girls was staffed by a matron and a cook who came only in the mornings. On the other hand, another of the same size had a matron, sister, relief staff nurse, full-time cook, night attendant and a part-time attendant. To a certain extent the niggardliness in the idea of what is required is due to the misconception to which reference was made in an earlier chapter—that is, that running a Home for people in care is little different from the running of an ordinary family home, where parents do not expect—or, if they do, find their expectations unfulfilled—to be relieved of their duties for stretches of each day. But the staff of a Home are not the parents or daughters of those they care for, and, moreover, the burden is never-ending. The work cannot be done properly unless the staff is sufficient to allow of regular free time and holidays.

16. According to our 'census' figures (see Chapter IV), staffing ratios vary widely, partly according to the type of resident in care, from an average of 1:10·3 in approved schools for boys to an average of 1:1·5 in residential nurseries. We had expected to find that there would be more staff in relation to the number of residents in small Homes than in larger ones, but the figures did not bear this out. In local authority children's Homes it was the very large establishments with over 100 children which had the highest number of staff in relation to children—1:3·5, whilst the smallest Homes, those with 10 children or less had a ratio of 1:3·8 which is close to the average for all children's Homes.

17. Similarly in local authority old people's Homes, it is the largest Homes where the staff ratio is highest, 1:5·1 in the largest compared with 1:5·6 in the smallest. But it is significant that the strain of work occasioned by lack of free time was stressed particularly by those working in small Homes and this points to understaffing.

18. It must be remembered too that staff ratios on paper are very different from the service available at any one time when illness, free time and holidays are taken into account. In Professor Townsend's survey of old people's Homes he quotes one example of a Home where there was a complement of 11 staff for 68 residents, but when allowance had been made for shifts off duty, holidays and so on there were never more than 4 people on duty at any one period during the day and 2 at

night.[1] In other words a paper ratio of 1:6 worked out in fact as 1:17 during the day and 1:34 during the night.

19. We are unable to recommend an 'ideal' staffing ratio, for there are too many variables to be considered. Great variety and flexibility are possible and to be commended. The lay-out of the Home, the physical frailty of the residents, the number of mentally infirm, the age of the children and their condition, the number of single rooms as opposed to dormitories, all these factors can influence the number of staff needed even when the total of residents is the same. There is scope for much research in this field. We draw attention in Chapter 10 to the help that could be derived from specific case studies and job analyses in determining the most economic use of our human resources.

20. But even without such detailed research we believe that much could be done to relieve staffs of some of the most onorous part of their long hours of duty. For example, in Homes catering for very frail elderly people, or mother and baby Homes where a girl may start her labour at any moment, the provision of good quality night staff probably does more to reduce the strain on the senior staff than anything else. (We have been told that in many areas there is not the same difficulty in recruiting night staff as day.) Regular relief staff during the day can be an advantage in other cases—people, that is, coming in regularly for a period to help with chores or to wheel out the babies in the afternoons. A trained nurse available for a group of Homes in one neighbourhood or a central pool of relief staff ready to go where needed during leave periods of the ordinary staffs are other methods that have been tried with success. In some areas it has been found best to attract help at the lower end of the hierarchy of staff and to 'upgrade' temporarily the rest of the staff. Not only is it often easier to maintain a relief pool of assistants than of more responsible people, but the temporary upgrading gives an added zest to those on the staff of the Home and acts as 'shadow training' for later promotion. In such circumstances it is, of course, essential that extra payment should be made for those taking the extra responsibility.

21. There are, again, many labour-saving devices that can be considered. When new Homes are built it is now usual to give a good deal of attention to these but even in older buildings much can be done, with a little thought, to reduce the energy and time spent on day-to-day chores. In too many Homes it is customary to assume that there is somebody ready to deputize for the cook when she is off duty and, in too many instances, the only person available is the matron. Experiments might be tried with the provision of deep-freeze, ready-to-heat

[1] *The Last Refuge*, op, cit., p. 77.

I

meals, such as are served on aircraft, an experiment already being tried in some hospitals. Such meals may be expensive, but so are cooks; and when the alternative is to over-burden people who are already working long hours, and so to cut down even further the number willing to undertake the job, such expenses may prove a very profitable investment.

22.   Comparatively few Homes are now so far from centres of population that it is difficult to get local women to come in as part-time workers and this provides a further source of relief. Unfortunately, in this, as in other occupations, there are some die-hards who refuse to face the realities of the present situation, and who accept only with the greatest reluctance the employment of part-time married women from the neighbourhood. Several witnesses spoke to us of 'being driven to temporary expedients like employing part-time staff'. It is necessary to realize that these are *not* 'temporary expedients' but an integral part of the contemporary scene. It is important because this affects the attitude to the part-time staff, the arrangements made for their comfort and the amount of teaching that one is prepared to give them about the duties demanded of them. It is worth noting that hospitals, schools and shops, all originally insisted that the work could not possibly be carried on efficiently with part-time workers and all have now come to depend on them as an essential part of their labour force. The same is true of residential establishments.

23.   Some witnesses have told us that the part-time staff are resented by the rest because they are unwilling to do the awkward shifts, in the evenings and at week-ends. On the other hand we have been given evidence that if it is made clear on appointment that some awkward hours are a condition of employment, it is usual for them to be accepted. Once workers have done a week-end duty and realized the need for round-the-clock care for residents, they often become sufficiently concerned for the welfare of those in their care to put their needs before their own. At the same time, it must be realized that the readiness to undertake such work depends to a great extent on the general labour situation of the locality. The more alternative part-time employments for women that are available, particularly if they are well paid and not unattractive, as in many highly industrial areas, the more difficult it is to recruit those who are willing to take duty shifts that interfere seriously with their own domestic obligations. In Northern Ireland, for example, where the percentage of unemployed is higher than in England and Wales, no difficulty at all is experienced in finding adequate numbers to do the awkward times. In the Midlands it is not so easy. Yet even there, if care is taken by those in charge to 'involve'

the part-time workers in the welfare of the residents, and if reasonable rotas are worked out, it is by no means impossible to attract suitable people.

24. Poor accommodation is often as great a hindrance to a reasonable private life as lack of free time. In many Homes that we have visited the needs of the assistant staff have been ignored, even when good and pleasant rooms have been provided for the Heads. It is unreasonable to expect the younger members of staff to entertain their friends or do their courting in a small sitting room which is the only place in which their colleagues can spend their off duty hours. Every resident worker should have at least a well-furnished bed-sitting room in which he or she is free—and has adequate space and equipment—to receive his own visitors, and where he can be sure of privacy. This need for an opportunity to have somewhere to call one's own—to be able to shut one's door—was constantly expressed to us. But the lack of proper accommodation is so great that there are many who feel compelled to leave the building altogether if they want to talk quietly to their own personal friends or to feel free of interruption.

25. We recognize that there are special problems in small children's Homes where children and staff live together in an intimate relationship and where it may be difficult to exclude children from staff quarters during free time. But even in normal family life the children are not made free of every corner of the house and must learn to accept that their elders occasionally prefer their room to their company. Being perpetually on the job and forever at the beck and call of those in care does not, in the long run, work for the good of the residents any more than of the staff. Too little time off, too few opportunities to let down one's hair leads to nervous strain and eventually to deterioration in the standard of service given.

26. There is still another side to this personal freedom. When people are living in a community there are certain adjustments that are essential for the convenience of all; but rules for the staff, as for the residents, should be kept to a minimum. Restrictions on guests, rules about lights out, times at which members of staff must come in at night and so on do not permit of a normal social, private life. For heads of Homes, the freedom to determine one's own leisure interests is generally taken for granted; but there are still too many Homes in which the younger members of staff do not enjoy similar privileges. There is no reason why young women should not come in late after dances or other evening entertainments, or receive their boy friends as they would in their own homes. Yet we came across one mother and baby Home where the managing committee has laid down regulations which not only insisted

that staff should be back at a very early hour after their free time but should not be permitted to let their boy friends come as far as the door-step of the Home. Such restrictions on personal liberty run counter to the whole climate of present day ideas and are likely to act as a very serious deterrent to recruitment of the kind of people needed for running the Homes.

27. It is still unfortunately true that there are employing bodies which expect too great a degree of dedication and self-sacrifice from those they employ; and since most of those who remain for any length of time in the work do so, at least partly, from a genuine desire to help those in need of care, there are large numbers who resign themselves to long hours of work, poor accommodation and exclusion from the normal social life of the neighbourhood. In some cases this is a matter of deliberate choice. Pioneers start experimental schemes and, 'with fire in the belly' are ready to devote themselves completely to their development. But it is not reasonable to expect all those engaged in the ordinary day-to-day running of Homes to show this single-minded self-sacrifice, nor would it be to the advantage of those in their care if they did. Although both local authorities and many volun-tary societies are fully aware of their responsibility to their staffs, there is, perhaps, a danger amongst some managing committees of assuming that those they employ in this humanitarian work need not expect the normal emoluments and conditions of employment, because this work should bring its own rewards and depends on charitable contributions. We believe this assumption to be unwarranted and harmful to the work they support.

28. Apart from privacy, what kind of accommodation should be provided? We believe that quiet well-heated bed-sitting rooms, flats or houses, with heating available during school vacations as well as term time, with facilities for some modest cooking and laundry, with storage space, and with bath and toilet amenities separate from those of the residents, are so obviously needed as hardly to need more than a mention. When we remember that 85 per cent of full-time care staff in children's Homes, and hostels for working boys and girls, 35 per cent of those in old people's Homes and Homes for physically handicapped adults and over 70 per cent in the other Homes are resident, it is clear that good accommodation must play a big part in life. 'Staff ought to have something nice to go home to' said the representatives of one voluntary organization to us. 'Their accommodation ought to be at least as attractive as their own home would be.' This does not mean that all members of staff want to retire behind a closed door on their evenings or days off. Far from it. Many told us how important they feel

it to be to share the lives—whether of children or others—for whom they are caring. The point we make here is that it should be a matter of choice and not of necessity. Even the most devoted and loving have their 'off' days and the accommodation provided should be such as to make it possible for them to be away from their charges when they wish. Our Census shows that even though a substantial majority of heads of Homes expressed themselves as satisfied with the accommodation provided for them, there was consistently less satisfaction with regard to privacy and personal cooking facilities than for any other facet of their lives.

29. Whatever may be the situation at the moment, the writing on the wall already points to the need for a radical re-consideration of this whole problem of accommodation. The changes in demographic trends and in marriage patterns discussed in Chapter V bring us face to face with a new situation. The single woman is rapidly disappearing from the labour market and there is no doubt that in the future we shall have to depend very much more than at present on married women returning to employment after a break to bring up their children, on married couples and on men. Many of these will have families of their own and the accommodation must take account of this. The children of staff members should not be compelled to share bedrooms with those in care, nor should a member of staff feel forced to resign because there is no room available for her child. Greater expenditure on staff quarters will be essential and, though bricks and mortar are not cheap, it may be money well spent. It is, to say the least, shortsighted to discourage continuity of staff because of unwillingness to invest in adequate facilities.

30. This brings us to an important question. Is it essential for the majority of the caring staff, in fact, to be resident? It is possible that, in the future, with the easing of the general housing situation and the increase in the proportion of married persons employed, even good accommodation will not attract a sufficient number of the kind of staff required. Indeed, we visited several Homes in different parts of the country where excellent staff accommodation had been empty for months because the staff preferred to remain in their own homes and come in daily for duty. For those with families, this is likely to be a growing trend. The time has come to give serious consideration to determining the proportion of those employed who *must* be resident and how far a high standard of care could be provided by non-residents.

31. First it is necessary to define what we understand by the terms. We have taken 'resident' to mean any situation in which it is obligatory for the staff to occupy the accommodation provided by the employing

body. This may not always be part of the main building; it may be a
self-contained flat within it, or there may be a separate staff wing or a
flat in the grounds. All these we consider to be 'residence'. By 'non-
residence' we imply that those employed live outside the curtilage,
usually in non-provided housing; or where the house is owned by the
employing authority, the use of it is not a condition of employment.
32. The majority of those who gave evidence to us assumed that this
work must be essentially resident for most of those employed. We
were continually told 'This is not a nine-to-five job' and 'There must
always be somebody in the Home to look after those in care'. We do
not question either of these statements, rather the contrary. But it may
be that the conclusions drawn from them are more the result of long-
standing practice and familiarity than of necessity.
33. We accept that some proportion of resident staff is essential
(though it should be stated that some of our members do not subscribe
completely to this view), but, in view of the difficulty of getting an
adequate number of suitable people willing to live in, it is important to
think clearly about the contribution that can be made by resident staff
and that could not be made by non-residents. We have come to the
conclusion that the benefits that stem from residence are two-fold. First
it is valuable to the sense of security and happiness of those in care that
there should be an individual who is identified as the 'caring' person;
and second, it is necessary for somebody to be readily available who is
competent to deal with an emergency. It is obvious that the first of
these is much more important than the second and particularly with
certain groups of people, as, for example, very young or disturbed
children, who gain help and confidence from the knowledge that the
person they trust is physically present and 'getattable'. Yet, as we have
argued earlier, even these people must have *some* time off and some
holidays if they are to keep their sanity. We came finally to the conclusion that in all the Homes within our terms of reference there should
be one person (or married couple) resident but that for the remainder,
residence should not be made a condition of employment. This does
not mean that there would be nobody on duty during the free times of
the resident person. There are already Homes in which non-resident
staff are provided with accommodation for certain nights of the week
when they are on duty and more could be done along these lines.
34. Our concern that more thought should be given to the need for
resident staff does not stem solely from difficulties of recruitment.
There is certainly no doubt that freedom from the obligation to live
in the Home would greatly widen the field from which potential staff
might be drawn; but we believe that it has also other advantages. Stress

has earlier been laid on the difficulty experienced by those who undertake this work in retaining the freshness of outlook and the broad interests that depend on constant contact with the general community and we believe that a Home staffed by a large proportion of those who come fresh each time to their tour of duty would find it much easier to become, and to remain, part of the neighbourhood than one in which the majority are so constantly involved that it is difficult for them to avoid developing into a closed community.

35. Some of our members feel so strongly that the future must lie mainly with non-resident staff that they have urged that experiments should be tried with completely non-resident staff. In old people's Homes, for example, they argue that there is no necessity for any member of staff to live there permanently, provided that there was some responsible person on duty throughout the whole day and night. We believe that there is here an area for careful experiment.

36. It should perhaps be made clear that we do not urge that staff should not be allowed to be resident. There are many people who prefer to live 'on the job' and indeed, the appeal of this kind of work consists largely in the opportunity it gives to humane and compassionate people to take responsibility for the comfort and happiness of those in need of care. It may even be that the lack of such opportunities might actually restrict recruitment instead of increasing it. But we believe that to a much greater extent than at present it should be a matter of individual choice and not a condition of employment.

37. The choice of 'living out' or 'living in' depends, of course, to a considerable extent on whether the Home is situated in an area in which other housing accommodation is available. Many people still think of the Homes within the scope of this report as consisting of a large mansion in the country. But this is not a true picture. Our Census returns show that few Homes are in isolated rural districts. In fact 84 per cent of all Homes are within twenty minutes walk of shops and 56 per cent are within twenty minutes walk of cinemas and other types of recreation. And most are on a good bus route. New Homes are almost invariably sited in or near an active community—for the sake of the residents as well as for the ease of getting staff. Yet there are some, particularly schools, and some Homes for old people, which are physically remote, and in such cases, it is almost impossible to get daily staff, whether as domestics or as those who 'care' for the people for whose benefit the Home is run.

38. But even where, as in the majority of cases, the Home is near a busy community—or in the middle of a newly built housing estate—the staff are often lonely and feel cut off from ordinary social life. One

must be careful not to over-emphasize this problem. On our group visits we were impressed by the number of people we met who were leading busy and enjoyable lives in the wider community and joining actively in the doings of clubs and churches. And we saw several Homes and schools which had obviously become a social centre for the neighbourhood—with the church or village fete held in the grounds, or the local youth club or old people's club meeting in their hall, and so on.

39.   Nevertheless there is a serious problem for many of those engaged in this work. Physical propinquity does not lead of necessity to social integration and care has to be taken that the Home does not become isolated from the locality in which it is situated. The officers of local authorities or central departments or of the headquarters of large voluntary organizations whose duty it is to visit Homes told us that even when the Home was sited in a busy housing estate, they spent the greater part of their visit simply listening to the members of the staff who were desperately anxious for somebody with whom they could talk. Such isolation leads to an 'ingrown' community, to petty grievances and bitter staff relationships. A sense of proportion is more quickly restored when the staff meet frequently with people whose interests, work and preoccupations are entirely different from their own. This is a two-way traffic; much can be done by managing committees and employing bodies to ensure that members of staff are invited to ordinary social occasions or to take part in the day-to-day activities of the locality. But there is also a responsibility on the staff to go half way to meet this, to be good neighbours to the housewives who live around and to welcome visitors, whether to the residents or to themselves. As far as the junior members of staff are concerned, the chief responsibility rests probably on the head of the Home who can make all the difference in the world to the speed with which people begin to feel themselves part of the local community. But the heads themselves, also need help in this connection. No Homes contain a cross-section of the community; they consist—apart from the staff—of old people, or handicapped persons, or children. It is an unreal life and this makes adjustment to other environments more difficult.

40.   Residents in an institution are even more liable to have emotional problems than people living independently. This creates a special problem for those who look after them. The concept of the 'therapeutic community', evolved in the care of the mentally ill, may be applicable in other residential institutions not intended for the mentally ill. The therapeutic community is one in which deliberate effort is made to use to the fullest possible extent, in a comprehensive treatment plan, the

contribution of all the staff and of all the patients. Each member contributes differently according to experience, needs and capacity. Those whose main experience seems to have been in suffering misfortune, may contribute most valuably by offering each other mutual support in evolving ways of understanding and coping with their troubles, and in helping the staff group to appreciate better what the needs are and how staff attitude, work and behaviour affect them. Doing this means opening up communications more fully than is usual. Staff and staff, staff and residents, residents and residents, are the communication links in mutual exchanges of ideas and attitudes which become part of the living community and change its nature. When communications are opened up like this there is much less likelihood of the residents feeling pushed around by 'Them', and they are more likely to appreciate staff problems and be more co-operative and make fewer unreasonable demands.

41. This concept of mutual exchanges is particularly appropriate to some kinds of residential care such as approved schools, but we think it would also be useful in, for instance, old people's Homes. If 'care' were more of a joint exercise between staff and residents, there might be less of that apathy among the old people which is so noticeable to the visitor to many old people's Homes.

42. It is sometimes said that the strains of living with your work are less for a married couple (or a matron or housemother with a husband working outside the Home) than for a single member of staff. Employing authorities have told us that the married matron is frequently more relaxed, whereas the single matron is 'always on the job'. But the married couple, particularly if they have their own children, have the extra strain of trying to maintain their own family life and yet be just to the claims the residents—old people or children—legitimately make on them; and this is likely to be especially difficult when the children are born in the Home. There may also be problems when staff and the residents in care come from different social backgrounds.

43. We believe that the kind of training we recommend in a later chapter will do much to help people to cope with these strains but there is also a need for much more support than is generally available at present. In the children's field something has been done by professional organizations such as the Residential Child Care Association to keep members of staff in touch with one another and by stimulating discussion of common problems reduce the feeling that one is alone in coping with 'a sea of troubles'. But the majority have not this help and solace. Their methods get out of date, their attitudes become more rigid and often enough they feel overwhelmed by the immensity of

their problems. Much could be done to relax this strain and by so doing add greatly to the value of the work that is done.

44. There should be frequent and regular meetings in an area so that those doing similar work can discuss their problems. Matrons on refresher courses usually show themselves so eager to talk to others with allied difficulties and gain so much by the knowledge that they are not alone and unique in the problems they encounter, that it is clear that they would eagerly welcome more opportunities for such exchanges of experience. There are many ways which might be suggested for the support that could be given to those who carry on this difficult work. In the past the lack of training for residential workers has sometimes created problems of communication between them and other professional workers; but if more are given the chance to take the kinds of training we describe in a later chapter we hope that this difficulty may be overcome. Frequent meetings organized by local authorities to enable their staffs and those of voluntary organizations engaged on related work in the locality to meet would be of value, so that those working in fairly small Homes could have the opportunity to learn—and to teach—others in the same field. Already this is done on a small scale by some authorities but a great expansion would earn real dividends in the stimulus and increased knowledge of those employed in this work. Regular refresher courses and visits from outside tutors to the Homes can be of enormous advantage because they help people who have got bogged down in an unending series of chores to step aside for a moment and try to see their work as a whole and in its context. In this respect there is need for the appointment of an Adviser (see also Chap. 7) to work with a particular group of Homes in an area. Most people, whatever their work, feel the need to talk over the special problems with which they are faced if they are to get, and keep, them in perspective. This is particularly important for residential workers because of the nature of the job. Most such workers feel, and with some justification, that outsiders do not appreciate the day-to-day problems of their close intimate relationship with difficult residents and to have the opportunity of constant discussion with an Adviser who, herself, had had experience in residential work would be of real value.

45. It is not within the scope of this report to discuss the relative advantages and disadvantages of Homes of different sizes. This is a matter of social policy. We are concerned only in so far as there are different staffing problems according to the size of the establishment. The problems to which we have drawn attention—social and professional isolation, inadequate free time and holidays, the restrictions on

private and family life and so on—are often more acute in the small Home than in the larger. Yet working in small Homes has its own satisfactions which appeal to those who enjoy the homely family atmosphere. This is probably more important in children's Homes where the house parents who have a small group under their care—often less than ten in number—can get to know them and love their individual characters in the intimate way usual in an ordinary family. They have too the pleasure of running their own little establishment in comparative independence.

46. But this has its dangers. Such a group is an artificial unit. Its numbers change and if many of the children stay only a short time the house parents may grow to feel like lodging house keepers. In such circumstances the burdens are more obvious than the satisfactions—the lack of privacy, the long hours, the difficulty of getting adequate time off, the problem of the relationship between one's own family and those in care and so on. The difficulty is greatest where the size of the Home allows for only one extra staff member other than the married couple in charge. It needs little emphasis to realize how lonely and vulnerable such an 'extra' may become.

47. In the old people's field it is rare to find Homes as small as some children's Homes; under 30 is generally counted as 'small', and the relationship is not necessarily as intimate as with the children. But here too it is more difficult to provide the number of staff that can ensure the constant needed care of the residents and yet give the conditions that we have earlier listed as essential. Yet is must be said that our Census shows a greater degree of stability in many of the smaller Homes than in the larger. In the small local authority children's Homes —that is, with 10 children or less—only 18 per cent of the assistant staff left annually compared with 33 per cent and over in every other size of children's Homes run by local authorities; and nearly two-thirds of the heads of these small Homes had stayed on the job for 5 years or more. In small local authority old people's Homes—that is, with under 16 residents—11 per cent of assistant staff left annually (about half as many as in the larger Homes) but in these the Heads showed a greater turnover. Nearly half of the local authority Homes with under 16 residents had had more than one head in 5 years, whilst for the larger Homes—with more than 30 residents—the proportion was about one-third.

48. It is clear that we need much more knowledge of the factors that combine to make a job satisfying to different kinds of people. Some enjoy the feeling that they are in charge and put up with the consequent disadvantages of lack of free time, privacy and rest. Others feel exactly

the opposite. As it is likely that there is a similar diversity in the likes and dislikes of people in care as of those looking after them, it appears that where possible the wisest course to follow would be to have a variety of different sizes so that residents could have the chance of fitting into the type of Home that suits them best as well as extending the field from which good recruits to the work could be chosen.

49. Salary scales are outside our terms of reference but the pay cheque is so important an incentive that we believe we ought to point out some of the existing factors in the situation which cause dissatisfaction. Over the field as a whole there is negotiating machinery to settle grades and rates of pay; but there is no national scale for assistant or deputy heads of Homes where these grades exist. At present this grade is one of the most difficult to fill and it is usual for those who take these jobs to show an exceptional rate of turnover. This is partly due to the fact already noted, that matrons tend to stay for several years so that deputies must move if they wish for promotion; but it is also due to the fact that local authorities pay very different rates and there is, therefore, a considerable amount of 'shopping around'. In one month the salaries advertised by different local authorities varied from £455 to £520 for a deputy head in a 60-bedded home to £840–£950 for a 50-bedded Home. Incidentally we may say that we do not accept the number of beds as the best criterion for determining salary scales. Size is not the only, or often the most, important measure of responsibility, and jobs which make heavy demands should carry extra pay, irrespective of the size of the Home. (See Chapter 7 for further discussion.)

50. One of the causes of dissatisfaction most frequently expressed to us was concerned with the charges made for board and lodging. When salaries are adequate it is reasonable to charge for food and accommodation and many of the staff appreciate that often excellent accommodation is provided at a cost far below its price in the market. But very often the amount deducted from salaries is the same whether the provision is good or bad. Those looking after children and sharing their lives pay as much as if they were given a private flat and even where some private room is offered, the same amount is deducted for a tiny bedroom at the end of a corridor as for a well equipped flat with all the normal amenities. We have also encountered staff sitting rooms which double as general offices, doctor's consulting room and an interview room for parents. We have already expressed our view of such inadequate provision. Here we make the additional point that if this is all that can be offered, it is not reasonable to make the same charge as if good rooms were available to the staff.

51. We have urged that residence should become more a matter of choice than it is at present. If this were so, we believe that there should be some difference between the rates charged for those who can choose whether to be residential or not and the rates charged for those for whom residence is a condition of employment.

52. Although the scales of salaries are not within our scope there are three matters to which we must draw attention. The first is that salaries of staff in Scotland as a whole compare unfavourably with those of their counterparts in England and Wales. In this connection we think it relevant to quote from the Report of the Secretary of State for Scotland on *Education in Scotland*, which, dealing with child care, states 'Probably the most important single reason for scarcity of staff is, however, that salaries and conditions of service generally compare unfavourably with those offered by some English local authorities. For this reason, the service in Scotland has lost some of its best staff, and has failed to recruit some able students trained in Scotland ... Until salaries and conditions of service are improved, it seems unlikely that the extended training arrangements ... will attract sufficient suitable staff to child care work in Scotland'.[1]

53. The second matter is the need to arrange salary scales in such a way as to encourage people to remain in the service for some considerable time. Experience has shown that the first years are the most vulnerable; the longer people stay in the job the more do their loyalty and affection grow. We believe that much could be done by more rapid increments in salary in early years and by the grant of a bonus after so many, say five, years of completed service. Such provision might prove most effective in tiding people over a period of uncertainty when they are undecided whether to remain or not. And it could be important as a financial recognition of years of service to those who do not become heads of Homes.

54. The third matter is the need to pay rates which can hope to attract the kind of men needed for these services. In Chapter 7 we point out that men have an essential part to play in residential work and urge that efforts should be made to employ an increasing number of them. This will be quite impossible unless the salaries bear some relation to those paid in other occupations which call for similar qualities and periods of training. It would be unfortunate if the only men who could afford to enter this field of employment were unmarried men or those with no family responsibilities.

[1] Report of the Secretary of State for Scotland on *Education in Scotland*, 1962 (Cmnd. 1975).

RECOMMENDATIONS

1. The practice already in force in some fields of care of limiting weekly hours of assistant staff to 40 should be extended. (Paras 8–10.)
2. As a minimum there should be provision for some free time each day. 1½ free days weekly and a long week-end every month. (Paras 11–13.)
3. Though the hours of senior staff cannot be rigidly laid down, staffing ratios should be calculated on a basis which allows a 40 hours week to be regarded as the norm. (Paras 9–10.)
4. Annual leave should be at least 4 weeks plus bank holidays (or time in lieu) and consideration should be given to allowing a longer period of leave after several years of service for those carrying heavy responsibility. (Para. 14.)
5. Free times and holidays should be arranged well in advance and should not be cancelled except for real emergencies. (Paras 5, 11.)
6. Consideration should be given to the possible uses and nature of relief staff and to the introduction of labour-saving arrangements. (Paras 20–23.)
7. Good accommodation should be provided for assistant staff as well as for those in charge. (Paras 24, 25, 28.)
8. Rules should be kept to a minimum and the staff allowed as much individual freedom as possible. (Paras 26–27.)
9. More experiments should be made into the greater use of non-resident staff. (Paras 30–36.)
10. More support should be provided for those in senior posts—by regular meetings, refresher courses and the appointment of an Adviser with experience in residential work. (Paras 38–44.)
11. As the size of Home affects the staffing problem there should be considerable diversity in size to suit the needs of different residents and give a range of choice to members of staff. (Paras 45–48.)
12. National salary scales for assistant (or deputy) matrons or heads of Homes should be negotiated. And for all staff more care should be taken to adjust the charges for board and lodging to the kind of provision made. (Paras 49–50.)
13. Salary scales should be arranged so as to provide an incentive to continue in service. (Para. 53.)
14. A bonus should be given for every 5 years of completed service. (Para. 53.)

7

RESIDENTIAL WORK AS A CAREER

PART I RECRUITMENT

1. The shortage of suitable men and women to staff the residential Homes is one of the serious factors in the present situation, for so many other problems—overwork, lack of regular free time, cancelled holidays, etc.—are directly connected with it. In this chapter, therefore, we consider the causes for this shortage and some of the ways in which recruitment might be encouraged.

2. There is no doubt that one of the deterrents to entering this occupation is the belief that its importance and skill are not recognized by the general public. As we pointed out in an earlier chapter there are, unfortunately, only too many people who think of it as no more than simply housework on a rather larger scale. This lack of status is not necessarily linked to the residential nature of the work but is much more closely allied to the lack of appreciation of the fact that this is a profession which requires specific training. It is significant that in the children's field, the status of the assistant staff in Homes run by the local authorities has risen appreciably since 1948 when the service and training for it were re-organized.

3. It is not only vis-à-vis the outside world that status presents its problems. Our evidence shows that house staff in many special and approved schools resent the fact that they are made to feel a wide gap between themselves and the teaching staff. There are, it is true, some schools which value them highly but many others are so 'teacher oriented' that the house staff feel themselves to be second class citizens. Quite apart from differences in salary and training, there are often irritating small discrepancies in treatment; for example, the use of separate sitting rooms.

4. Other professions have started with a similar handicap but have overcome it. When Florence Nightingale first sent her 'lady nurses' into the hospitals they entered an occupation that had depended on the

lowest grades of unskilled women workers, and the main incentive
to the recruitment of the kind of woman she was determined to get was
primarily her insistence on training. The gulf between the 'lady nurse'
and Mrs Gamp was the gulf between the trained and the untrained.

5. Every profession as it emerges is characterized by the training
which it prescribes. The full case for training is set out in Chapter 8
but its importance in improving the image of the occupation must not
be overlooked. If the courses offered are of sufficient intellectual content to compare with the training already available for other kinds of
work, such as teaching, nursing, social work and so on, residential
work will come to be accepted by young men and women when
choosing their careers, and by their parents, as one amongst other
alternative and acceptable fields of employment.

6. To some extent the ideas about residential work lag behind the
facts. In a good Home it is neither so onerous nor so underpaid as it
used to be, and there are substantial material rewards to add to the
satisfactions of doing a worth while job. But the salary levels and, in
particular, the deductions for board and lodging make the men and
women employed in this work *feel* less well paid than others of their
acquaintance. We live in an affluent society and the rates of pay of
most occupations are much higher than they used to be, but we must
remember that costs of living also continually rise and thus the emoluments enjoyed by residential workers become consequently more and
more valuable. Nevertheless most of them are inclined to underestimate this because they are not faced with the task of making their
daily household purchases for themselves and so do not easily recognize
the inroads on the higher payments received by others.

7. But there are two factors which do, undoubtedly, play a real part
in any comparison with the remuneration earned in other spheres. The
first is the fact that the amount charged for board and lodging does not
bear any close relation to the accommodation and amenities offered and
what may be a small price to pay in one Home may be serious over-
payment in another. The second is, that the worker in residence does
not exercise the same amount of individual choice as those whose home
life is separated from their work. It may be that the increase in the
proportion of non-resident staff in the future, which we discussed in the
previous chapter, may lessen this problem.

8. There are some who believe that the present lack of an acceptable
terminology, to which reference was made in the first chapter, is a
further hindrance to recruitment. Most of our witnesses felt that such
names as 'house father' or 'house mother' are distinctly non-glamorous
and that young people, in particular, are rather repelled by the thought

that they may be so designated. As far as heads of Homes are concerned it might be helpful if the term 'head of Home' or 'officer in charge' could be used solely as a description of the post (for advertisements, for example, or for salary negotiations) whilst those filling such posts were always referred to by their names as Mr X or Miss (or Mrs) Y.

9. In present practice the second in command is usually, but not invariably, called the Assistant or Deputy . . . (according to the name given to the head). It is probable that the term Deputy would prove more attractive as well as being, in fact, a more correct description. We do not feel ourselves able to make any firm recommendations on terminology but we recognize that it is well worth serious thought.

10. In most occupations those who enter have a fairly clear picture of future possibilities that may be open to them. They are aware of posts which carry wider interest, greater responsibility and higher remuneration than those of the beginner. But in residential work there is no clear career structure beyond a rather limited point. The substitution of a large number of small Homes for a few of greater size does, indeed, provide many more opportunities to become the head of a Home, but after this there are mot many possibilities of further promotion. We realize that the chance of rising to higher posts is not of equal importance to all sections of this occupation. There are many people who are attracted to it because their domestic obligations demand that they look for work in their own neighbourhood and they are content to do a satisfying job, so long as the conditions of employment are suitable, without any thought of promotion. And there are also many others who even though they are not limited in this way are content to continue with the kind of work they find worthwhile and do not wish to move to further responsibilities.

11. But there is no doubt that there is a considerable proportion who are anxious to move forward as their knowledge and experience grow. All these categories of worker are important. There will always be a great need both for the locally recruited and for those whose ambitions do not soar too high; but it is also very important to attract those whose abilities and interests would fit them for supervisory posts, and it is with this group that we are here principally concerned. It is only if we can offer the likelihood that more rewarding posts will be available as knowledge grows (rewarding both in interest and remuneration) that men and women of ability will be willing to enter this occupation.

12. We have spoken of the acute staff shortage, yet our census figures show that over the whole field only about 5 per cent posts are vacant at any one time and only 2 per cent are vacancies of long standing. The apparent contradiction is explained by the fact that most employing

K

authorities feel compelled to fill their posts however unsuitable they know the applicants to be. 'Recruiting for old people's Homes is catch as catch can' said one witness and as another said to us, 'We have put up with the mediocre for fear we get the incompetent in their place'. And yet even so it is only after repeated advertisement that most posts are filled.

13. The poor quality of some recruits results in a very high labour turnover. As the Census shows, 28 per cent of assistant staff leave every year, so that not only are employing bodies faced with the need to recruit over one quarter of their staff anew each year, but the heads of Homes have the task of teaching this large proportion of their assistants every year afresh.

14. The seriousness of the situation cannot be overestimated, for it is certain to increase, rather than diminish in importance, unless drastic changes are made. The residential service will need a large number of people because of the increased number of places which must be provided in the next ten years; and it needs a better qualified staff because the job is constantly becoming more skilled and more exacting for the reasons to which we have several times drawn attention in other chapters.

15. We believe that the better conditions of employment which we have recommended in Chapter 6 and the training schemes which we outline in Chapter 8 are not only of value, and indeed essential in themselves, but that they would have an altogether favourable impact on the recruitment of the numbers and kinds of men and women who are needed for this work. But at the same time we have to face the fact that there is keen competition from other occupations, and that the pool of labour in which the residential service has been accustomed to fish is no longer so large nor so well stocked as it used to be.

16. We are still depending to a great extent on the unmarried women who have for so long been the backbone of the service. As the Census shows, one-third of the women currently employed in Homes are over 50. But in the future we cannot depend on this pool of labour. Whereas 15 per cent of those women who were born in the first decade of this century remained single, the changes in birth and marriage rates are such that now about 5 per cent of young women will remain unmarried. Not only this but they marry at an earlier age. This is the stark fact that must be faced. All the occupations that have depended on single women must now recognize the new situation, and it must be realized that so far as residential work is concerned this is especially serious, for it also affects the numbers available for the nursing services on which so far residential work has depended to a great extent.

17. We must cast our net more widely and be ready to change many of our old ideas if we are to get the numbers of suitable people who are needed. Where should we look for this supply?

18. First we can hope to attract more young people if we are prepared to offer good training, reasonable conditions of employment and the possibility of a career in the future. At present the many young women who are drawn to work in this field before their marriage go into children's Homes but there is no reason why they should feel themselves restricted to this section. In several European countries a high proportion of those who work in Homes for old people are young women; they seem to enjoy it and they certainly give a good deal to the old people for whom they care. In this country only 2 per cent of the 'caring' staff in old people's Homes are under 21. Is this small proportion necessary or is it simply the result of habit?

19. One of the encouraging facts of the present employment situation is the widespread interest of those leaving school at sixteen or seventeen, amongst girls especially, who wish to do work which enables them to give service to people. The evidence for this comes from a number of sources: from enquiries to employing bodies; from careers conferences and from all varieties of schools. It is possible that, in some instances, this is only a passing phase and is part of the general 'climate' of adolescence; but for many it develops into a lasting interest, and is likely to do so in more cases if residential care offers more training and better prospects than at the moment. It is unfortunately true that only too often the generous enthusiasm of young people is killed by the reception they receive. Either they are told to 'do something else for a while until they are more mature' or, if they are accepted, they are confined to routine and uninteresting chores. As a rule we accept that both girls and young men should be at least 18 before they can be expected to have enough experience of life to start work or training in a residential setting. In modern children's Homes which include boys and girls of varying ages, young members of staff may be considered too nearly of the same age group as their charges to be given any responsibility. And the limitations imposed by hours of work and so on may cut them off too much from the enjoyments and experiences of their contemporaries in other kinds of work. But all these objections would be less cogent if the changes we recommend for the future take place. With a larger proportion of non-resident staff there would be more opportunity for the younger age group who could continue their education and share the normal activities suitable to their age just as much in this occupation as in any other.

20. We hope that the scheme of training for those over 18 will offer

an incentive to more young people, but there are many other ways in which even those below this age can come to think of it as one of the alternatives to consider when they are contemplating their working lives. Carefully arranged opportunities for older schoolchildren to do regular work in local Homes; reading aloud or preparing the tea once a week for old people, helping in a children's Home, are obvious ways of harnessing the eagerness to do something that is worth while that is, happily, so marked a characteristic of youth; jobs which are helpful at the moment and which also open the eyes of young people to what is entailed in the care of others. Youth Employment Officers would certainly be more willing to help recruit young people if they could be assured that they would not be exploited either emotionally or simply as an extra pair of hands. When training is provided and pretraining work is available to give those interested a taste of the job, it is fairly certain that the Central Youth Employment Executive would be ready to give much wider publicity to residential care as an opening for young people.

21.   As things are at present, the majority of those in residential work are women and this emphasis is particularly marked in the younger age groups. As most girls are now married and beginning their families by the early twenties, the young people who may be attracted in the ways we have suggested will leave the occupation after a few years. But this does not mean that they are lost forever. It is now becoming common practice for women to return to paid employment when their most pressing domestic obligations are over and those who are willing to re-enter this field at 35-45 have 20 to 25 years of service to offer. The more care that has been given to the training and suitable employment of girls between leaving school and marriage, the greater likelihood that those who leave to marry will be ready to come back for the second phase of their employment. But the older women we should like to recruit are not confined to those who have had experience of residential work in their early years. Whatever the kind of work that may have been done before marriage, the more mature woman is needed. Bringing up a family is the kind of experience that can make an excellent foundation for the training that is necessary for residential work; and the probability that those entering during their thirties or forties are likely to remain in the job makes it eminently worth while for them to be offered such training.

22.   Thirdly we must look to married couples. In some cases it may be that it is the wife who is appointed whilst the husband continues to pursue his own occupation; in others a joint appointment may be possible. Some employers have told us that they find it preferable to

employ only one partner, whilst providing accommodation for both and any children they may have, because it is not easy to find married couples both of whom are equally suited to the work; others, on the contrary have said that they prefer both to be in the work because each can contribute so much and their joint interest makes them more stable and more relaxed. This is a matter on which it is impossible to generalize. Probably all the employers who gave us their views based their opinions on the experience they happened to have had.

23. The view has sometimes been expressed to us that there is not enough work, other than assistance with the general administration, for a man to feel that he is pulling his weight. We are anxious to make it clear that we do not think of men in this work as merely 'half a married couple'; they have a very real and important role of their own to play.

24. In approved or special schools for boys or in a boys' hostel there is an obvious and satisfying role for men to fill, for this is a normal part of a boy's education. In Homes for the old and the mentally disordered and the socially inadequate there is also a place for men to help with their care and to encourage suitable activities. In children's Homes the absence of a male figure impoverishes a child's experience. At one time there was strict sex segregation in children's Homes and many grew up without ever having the opportunity to establish friendly relations with a grown man. This has changed and with the present emphasis on mixed Homes, men and women co-operate in the family life. Children need the influence of both men and women in their lives. For a girl of school age the presence of men as a normal part of the social pattern is essential if she is to develop the understanding of the parts played by men and women in the world; and there are many play activities in which the man's contribution can be outstanding. Hiking, exploring, camping, hill-climbing, a host of 'do-it-yourself' jobs can help children to learn to act independently and to expand their mental and spiritual horizons. In the normal family the father is as much a part of a child's realization of the world as the mother; in the substitute home, the presence of a man is equally necessary. This is just as true of the approved schools and special schools for girls as for boys.

25. We have, at the same time, to be realists. We recognize that there are difficulties to be met in the selection of the right kind of man, particularly, perhaps, in dealing with disturbed children. And it is also likely that the very young man may not be able to contribute much in a residential post until he has had some experience of life. But with the increasing shortage of young women, due to earlier marriage, all occupations which up to now have relied almost exclusively on female

labour, will have to learn to recruit more men. For residential work we think it important to try to attract more men, not only because they are less likely to 'waste through marriage' but because we believe that they have a positive contribution to make.

26. There are two further points we wish to make about recruitment. First, the use of those with nursing qualifications. We believe that residential Homes should not deliberately try to recruit nurses unless they are definitely needed for medical reasons. There is a serious shortage of nurses for the work they are specially trained to do and they should not be drawn away for other work which does not require their particular expertise. When nursing is needed only incidentally, as in most Homes, it can be provided in other ways, either by local authority nursing services or by daily visits from a nurse living in the area. Some nursing skill will also be taught in the syllabus for training courses for residential care staff. This does not mean, of course, that nurses should be prevented from entering residential care work if they wish. This should be, as are all matters of occupational choice, something that the individual has the right to settle for herself. But if a nurse does wish to undertake residential care work she should be expected to take the appropriate course of training. A nursing qualification is not a substitute for this.

27. The second is the valuable contribution that can be made by overseas staff. Some who are already trained come over for two or three years to learn English and then return to their own countries. Others come with the idea of making this their permanent home. Both groups should be welcomed for the part they can play.

28. So much for the people whom we can hope to attract into residential work; but there is need for a better system than exists at present for bringing together Homes in need of staff and suitable persons willing to work in them. The most usual way of recruiting senior supervisory staff at present is by advertisement in newspapers and such weekly journals as the *British Hospital and Social Service Journal,* the *Times Educational Supplement, New Society,* the *Lady* and others. Little has been done to try to establish which periodicals are more likely to bring responses and most managing committees seem to make haphazard choices. Certainly a good deal of money is wasted in this way and advertisements are constantly repeated even though no answers at all are received or only from entirely unsuitable people.

29. Much could be done to improve this situation. For example it is evident that some people prefer to work for local authorities and some for voluntary bodies so journals should be asked to classify their advertisements accordingly. Again the layout of many advertisements

is deplorable and it is probable that they would be more likely to catch the eye and arouse interest if several posts were advertised simultaneously instead of a series of small type announcements that can easily be overlooked.

30. Many of our witnesses felt that more use might be made of the mass media to show the nature of residential work. Frequent references were made to the success that was thought to have resulted from TV programmes such as those on Foster Parents Employment Offices, and voluntary agencies such as the Citizens Advice Bureau, the W.R.V.S. and the Red Cross would almost certainly be willing to distribute literature if it were obtainable; and when training courses are available the Colleges of Further Education will become valuable centres of information. But also the value of personal contacts and experience must not be underestimated. According to the Home Office Survey 16 per cent of current staff learned of the existence of the job through direct personal experience in a children's Home, 43 per cent learned indirectly through friends, 18 per cent through television and newspapers and 12 per cent through such official sources as the Ministry of Labour, the Home Office, schools etc. The large part thus shown to be played by personal contact is confirmed by the evidence of many matrons whom we saw who had 'happened' into residential work by accident; they had heard of the job through the C.A.B. or the Vicar or through doing voluntary work for the W.R.V.S. or a similar organization.

31. We cannot leave this question of the ways in which responsible posts may be made known without urging that in future no advertisement should appear, as happens so often at present, which includes the words 'no experience necessary'. We recognize the despair which leads to such action. Nevertheless it can do nothing but harm—in attracting unsuitable people, in lowering the status of the work and in spreading the fallacious idea that this is not skilled work but can be undertaken without preparation by anybody.

32. Whatever the media for making known vacant posts, advertisements should be accurately worded and set out clearly the terms of appointment. Replies to applicants should be prompt and courteous and references should always be taken up before interviews are held. (We stress this last point because it is often ignored. One of the largest organizations in the field of child care told us that when members of their staff leave to go into other residential work they are asked for references in only about 10 per cent of cases. In this way, quite unsuitable people can go on for years from job to job, doing untold damage.)

33. During interviews with applicants we believe that care should be

taken not to paint too rosy a picture of the work. Indeed, more success is likely if the work is represented as a challenge and not as something easy. It is better for applicants to know what is entailed from the start and witnesses have told us that the better candidates are rarely put off by knowing the difficulties as well as the satisfactions of the work. The Home Office Survey shows that only 14 per cent of house mothers and 21 per cent of assistants had been warned during their interviews of parts of the work which they later found unpleasant. Many complained that they had much more housework to do and less time to spend with the children than had been anticipated. Such sins of omission can quickly lead to disillusion and a heavy labour turnover.

34.   Wherever possible, an applicant should not be appointed without a visit to the Home or one which is very similar. The Home Office Survey said that 40 per cent were offered a post without being taken round any children's Home at all.

35.   Selection of staff is never an easy task, but it cannot be well done unless the selectors themselves are well informed about the nature of the work to be performed. This means not only that the appointing body should understand what the jobs require in the way of administrative, nursing, domestic or social skills but that they should be clear on the role of the particular post they are anxious to fill. For example, it is not unusual for those responsible for old people's Homes or mental hostels to appoint a nurse because they are aware of particular problems to be solved and then later assume that the person selected is equally capable of performing entirely different skills. It is no wonder if, in such circumstances, the person who accepts the post is confused about what she is really expected to do.

36.   We are strongly of the opinion that all appointments should be subject to a probationary period on both sides. The only way in which the capacity of staff can be assessed is in the working situation, not during the interview where future performance can only be conjectured. And similarly the applicant cannot be sure how she will fit into the pattern of the Home until she has had some experience of the others in the group with whom she will have to work in close collaboration. If appointments were made for a probationary period of so many months it would be simpler for both parties to terminate an unsatisfactory situation.

37.   It seems clear to us that so much of the difficulty of recruiting people for this work is due to ignorance that there is a need for some centre of information. We do not think of this as an employment agency, advertising posts or conducting preliminary interviews. We are convinced that most employing bodies prefer to carry out these

functions themselves. But there should be one place to which those interested could apply for accurate and up-to-date information on all aspects of the work; e.g. the different sections of the occupation, the qualities and qualifications required, the courses of training available, the rates of pay and general conditions of employment, where to look for choice of vacancies, the prospects of promotion and so on.

38. For some time a service of this kind has been advocated for the field of social work and a Social Work Advisory Service has been recently set up under the auspices of the Standing Conference of Organizations of Social Workers. It is to be administered by an independent charitable trust and is financed by a generous grant for an initial three years from the Calouste Gulbenkian Foundation. The service is intended to provide information about education and training for social work and career prospects; give individual advice to applicants; and provide links with other organizations in this field. Such a development would do much to help the residential field. It is possible that the Social Work Advisory Service might consent to take this under its own wing; if this did not prove possible, the central training body for residential work which we recommend might undertake this as one of its duties.

PART II: THE PROSPECTS OF THE JOB

39. We turn now to residential work from the point of view of its prospects as a career. What is the present position? The larger number of smaller Homes compared with twenty years ago has created many more head and deputy head posts, so that nowadays a large proportion can expect to get work of considerable responsibility a short time after entering the service. But the career structure is a short ladder with few rungs. In old people's Homes the usual establishment consists of assistants (or attendants) senior assistants, sometimes an assistant matron, then a deputy matron and matron. In practice it is unusual for those who begin as assistants to climb up the ladder to the post of matron, not because of any unwillingness on the part of employing authorities to promote but because of the many factors which operate to separate the grade of assistants from that of the senior staff. A very large number of assistants are local residents who are prepared to do this work because it fits in well with their own domestic obligations. It is the convenience of the job rather than the appeal of the particular type of work which is the main inducement. Few of them think of the work as a long-term career and even though they are glad to help in work which satisfies their eagerness to do something which contributes

to the welfare of others, the nature of the job is generally subordinate to their individual and family interests. Most of them are non-resident and their salaries and conditions of service are quite distinct from those of the senior staff. Their hours are fixed and they are paid for overtime. The promotion of assistants to assistant or other matron grades is therefore rare and, indeed, an assistant who was thus promoted might find herself with more responsibility, longer hours of work without overtime payment, and thus a smaller weekly pay packet.

40. In children's Homes recent social policy has resulted in a very large number of small Homes (much smaller than the 'small' Home for old People) so that there are better chances of being appointed a house mother than used to be the case, but the only opportunity of promotion for the woman in charge of a small family group Home is to be moved to a larger one. In larger Homes there are usually an assistant house mother, house mother, deputy head and head, but it is less usual for a single woman to be offered the position of head of a mixed home, as authorities prefer to appoint a married couple. Men who have taken suitable training are often attracted from children's Homes into approved and special schools partly because their prospects may be brighter in these fields and partly because of the interest of working with a team of other professional workers.

41. How readily people can move from junior to senior appointments seems to vary with different employing bodies. In a local authority's children's department there is often quick promotion for junior staff who show ability, but fewer vacancies and less movement for senior staff. One very large authority told us that few heads of their Homes had risen from their own junior ranks; but on the other hand, a large voluntary organization said that 64 per cent of their heads had been promoted from amongst their own employees.

42. In approved and special schools there is less chance for house staff to become heads of establishments; the primary purpose of schools is educational and the top posts generally go to teachers. But as far as the approved schools are concerned, with a growing realization of the importance of social education and the contribution made by house masters and mistresses, there is less certainty that the headship must be held by a teacher.

43. In the remainder of the field the hierarchy is similar but the ladder is even shorter. In many small Homes there is often nobody but the matron and her assistant apart from the domestic workers, and no prospect of further promotion. There are certain institutions which are doing especially interesting experimental work or which have gained a wide reputation, which are able to attract capable people who can

generally move on to other jobs because employers are anxious to have staff with this special experience. But these are exceptions. In most residential work, whilst there is a reasonable prospect for competent people to become the heads of Homes, it is much more difficult to go further.

44. We want to make it clear that we do not assume that everybody in this, any more than in any other occupation, is vitally concerned with promotion. Indeed it is possible that the proportion of those in residential work who want to move up the ladder is less than in many other spheres. Many heads of Homes are content to remain as they are 'To look after 60 old people properly and run a Home well is a most sophisticated and difficult social job and one which pays unbelievable dividends' said one head to us and this sentiment was echoed by many others. Yet however rewarding the majority may feel the work to be, there are others who are aware that they have capacities for which there is no outlet and it is important that the service should attract these if it is to have the leadership it needs.

45. There are, no doubt, many young people who are attracted to the work solely out of generous motives and without much thought for the future. Nevertheless a time may come later on when they begin to be aware that their contemporaries in other occupations have risen to posts of responsibility and higher status and feel resentful that they have no similar opportunities. We believe that we should concern ourselves with their prospects even if they do not do so themselves at the outset of their employment. But, as we have seen, these are not the main body of workers, for the majority of young women are unlikely in any case to remain in the work without a break and the older and more experienced women who enter an occupation to which they may possibly devote 20 to 25 years are much more likely to be concerned about the prospects it offers. At least some proportion of them will wish to prepare themselves—either by the one year course for mature students or by other means—for senior posts. Nor is it likely that many men will be attracted to this work unless there are long term prospects open to them which compare, both in responsibility and material rewards, with those available in comparable occupations.

46. For all these reasons therefore we believe it essential to try to map out possible lines of development. One of the things we are anxious to avoid is to give the impression that the only way to promote those who have shown themselves especially highly skilled in residential work is to offer them jobs which take them out of it; but there are many ways in which the knowledge and experience they have gained may be used in supervisory and advisory posts which are still within the residential service.

47. First, the training courses which we recommend will demand a number of tutors who themselves have had experience in the field. We believe that most of these tutors should be based on the educational establishment where the courses will be held, but they will go into Homes both in connection with work done by students as part of their training and to help heads of Homes to organize in-service and staff development training for all the members of their staff. This dual function will demand capacity of a high order.

48. Second, there is the consultative work to be done. Any organization which is responsible for a number of Homes, whether it is a local authority or a large voluntary organization, must employ people to visit the Homes in order to ensure that they are run in accordance with the policy laid down and to advise those doing the work. In one sense this might seem to be the function of an inspectorate but in practice it is very much more an advisory and consultative service. Here again is an interesting and rewarding form of work for senior staff and this is likely to be particularly so when those in charge of Homes will have had a comprehensive course of training as well as years of experience.

49. In an earlier chapter we stressed the need for more supportive persons to break down the professional isolation in which so many heads of Homes find themselves, and to provide opportunities for those in different Homes to pool their experiences. The Advisers whose appointment we recommend are unlikely to be either the sympathetic listeners required or able to offer constructive advice to those they visit unless they themselves have had considerable experience in the work. This kind of post already exists in some areas and in a good many voluntary organizations but it is capable of great expansion with advantage to the service. Here again is another possible avenue for promotion.

50. All the forms of work so far enumerated make direct and fruitful use of the knowledge and experience gained in residential work and, indeed, could not be done adequately by those who have not had actual experience in Homes. But there are also possibilities of more purely administrative posts which may prove attractive to some. The work of running a large Home or group of Homes with all its problems of budgeting, arranging staff duties and developing good staff relations gives opportunities for the exercise of administrative skills and many may welcome the chance of moving over into administrative work in the local authorities or voluntary organizations connected with residential work.

51. We believe too that promotion should sometimes take the form of a higher recognized status in the same job. There is room for credit

to be given for exceptional work by a higher salary scale without the necessity for moving from a post in which the great experience that has been gained has the best chance of being of value.

52.   In the first chapter we asked ourselves the question, 'Is residential work a single profession or is it a number of related ones?' We have given careful thought to the possibility of creating a common career structure for all residential work so that people could move freely from one branch of work to another. If this were possible it would open many more opportunities for rising to posts of greater responsibility than exist at the moment. Even now the lines of demarcation are not completely watertight. There is some movement from one type of work to another, e.g. from children's Homes to approved schools; the Royal College of Nursing told us that nurses often move from caring for children to caring for old people, and evidently, with success; and the Methodist Homes for the Aged have employed several members of staff who had earlier been working in children's Homes and have experienced no difficulties in making the transition.

53.   Many witnesses said that older people find it increasingly difficult, after some years, to offer children the same intimate relationship that younger people can; and most agree that it is not generally wise to have too wide an age gap between children and those caring for them. It might seem that many workers would welcome a change of scene and charge and that, following the pattern in ordinary family life, those who find satisfaction in looking after children or young people in their own early years might prefer to care for older people later on.

54.   Yet we are bound to admit that when we put this point of view to our many witnesses it did not generally meet with acceptance. We were continually told that those who go into this work have extremely definite predilections and that they would be more likely to leave the field altogether than to move to another section of it. There are some who feel themselves drawn to look after children, others who want to care for the old, and others again to find satisfaction in helping the handicapped, or mother and babies and so on.

55.   Nevertheless we ask ourselves if this attitude is as unchangeable as it was sometimes described to us as being. In most instances our question came as a surprise to our witnesses; it was a suggestion that had not before entered their minds because, for various reasons, the different kinds of work are so separate in their organization and control that they had taken it for granted that their work lay in one special direction. To a certain extent, then, their answers may have been simply the reaction to any, seemingly, revolutionary idea. It is impossible for us to judge how far this may have been the case and how far these

boundaries represent unsurmountable barriers between the different parts of the same field.

56.   We feel convinced, however, that however strong these barriers may be at the moment, they are likely to be very much lessened by the forms of training we have recommended. The common basis for all the courses we envisage before any specialization begins, has been proposed on purely educational grounds; but at the same time, we think that it may lead to a much greater recognition than is usual now of the close relation between all forms of work which are based on caring for human beings in a residential setting. If this has the result we hope for, that those entering the field of residential care begin to think of it as one profession with many specialisms instead of as a number of separated types of work, the opportunities for advancement of those who wish to have a continuous career in it will be very materially increased.

57.   This changed concept of residential care as one profession can have little hope of development unless employing authorities realize the necessary alterations in terms of employment that it demands. It would be idle, for example, to expect people to be prepared to move from work with a local authority to work with a voluntary organization if this involved them in a serious loss of pension rights. But this is now a universal problem. In industry and commerce we are belatedly beginning to realize that the most efficient deployment of our human resources cannot be effected if people are bound to a particular kind of job by the knowledge that mobility will result in a loss of superannuation and other rights which are not interchangeable. Employing bodies in the residential field in common with all other employers will have to be ready to alter their conditions of service to meet the needs of the times.

RECOMMENDATIONS

1.   The shortage of staff at present and the likelihood of increased demands in the near future makes it essential to find new sources of recruitment; e.g. older women, more men and married couples (Paras 16-25).

2.   Consideration should be given to the organization of pre-training work for young people (Paras 19-20).

3.   More care should be taken in the framing and distribution of advertisement of posts (Paras 28-32).

4.   The methods of selecting and appointing candidates for posts should be improved (Paras 33-36).

5. A central Information Office should be established, preferably in connection with the new Social Work Advisory Service (Paras 37–38).

6. A carefully organized career structure should be formulated (Paras 44–51).

7. Steps should be taken to facilitate the movement of workers from one kind of residential work to another (Paras 52–57).

8

TRAINING

1. The essence of training is to inculcate principles, provide a background of knowledge, develop skills, and encourage the student to regard learning as a continuous process to be undertaken throughout his subsequent career. Clearly no training can equip him to meet every eventuality he will encounter on the job, but it should give him some acceptable basis for thought and action. The question of training has therefore inevitably become one of our main areas of concern.

2. In the residential field, in which there are few trained workers, recruitment has inevitably been difficult. Though the local standing of those in charge may be high, the general status of residential work is undoubtedly low. Yet the work involved is increasingly difficult and responsible. Residential establishments, which get more and more costly to maintain, should be rightly used. They are no longer expected simply to provide custodial care and shelter. Children and adults are in them because skilled care in a residential setting is needed and is of a nature that cannot be provided elsewhere. Staff therefore require more knowledge and insight for their job if it is to be done properly. They are making an important—indeed a unique—contribution because they are called upon to help people who cannot be helped so effectively in any other way. Today adults in residential establishments are likely to have either serious physical or mental handicaps, or be of considerable age and infirmity; whilst many of the children will be so handicapped or disturbed in their behaviour that they need skilled remedial care. Moreover the staff should often have regard not only to the needs of individual residents, but to working constructively with their relatives and friends.

3. To do such difficult work satisfactorily, staff need personal qualities such as warmth and imagination, but clearly they should also be given the opportunity to equip themselves through adequate training. Indeed to expect them to undertake such work without this is fair neither to them nor to the people for whom they are

caring. Experience is essential; but unless it is reinforced by training it cannot provide knowledge, understanding and skill which are equally vital.

4. The need for training for residential work has long been recognized in the field of child care. Although it may seem extremely ambitious to advocate a full-time training course to include workers in all other fields, we are convinced that unless this is provided the level of the work carried out solely on the basis of experience will increasingly fall short of requirements, while the problem of staffing residential establishments will become even more serious in the future than it is at present.

5. Five main resons stand out for providing training for residential work. Firstly, training gives increased understanding of the reasons for the behaviour of children and adults, and a knowledge of ways in which their needs may be met. Secondly, it can help students to apply this knowledge to themselves, so that they may become aware of their own feelings and motives. Residential workers need this awareness because their attitude and values will determine the kind of assistance they are able to give to those in their care. Training should help them to acquire insights which will enable them to use personal relationships effectively in their work. Thirdly, training can give knowledge and understanding of the problems and opportunities of life in a residential group. A group is something more than the sum total of the individuals that make it up, and the behaviour of individuals is affected by the relationships and pressures that exist within it. Staff as well as residents have to learn to live as a group, and training can help in this process. Fourthly, training widens the horizons of residential staff by giving them some knowledge of the social services and an appreciation of the place of residential establishments within the total social provision, thus helping such staff to work with the relatives of the residents and with doctors, social workers and others as members of a service with common interest and purpose. Lastly, our evidence shows that those already in the work are well aware of the need for a comprehensive training plan, which would be likely to attract a quality of entrant who might be held back because of the lack of such provision in most of the fields we have examined.

6. Some alternatives to a full-time course were suggested at various times by our witnesses. It has been said, for instance, that skills in residential work cannot be taught outside the residential setting and therefore the only training offered should be in-service training. We fully accept that practical experience in residential settings would be an essential element in any scheme of training and recognize the value

L

of informal discussions with staff and fellow students. Nevertheless we are convinced that only a well-designed full-time course, which combines systematic teaching with practical illustrations and experience, would provide students aiming to hold responsible jobs with a sufficient opportunity for learning and the stimulation which they require. An exclusively on-the-job training is quite inadequate for such a purpose.

7. Another solution presented was for a 'sandwich' type of course for the older entrant, with periods of paid employment alternating with attendance at a course centre. In other fields, as for example industry, such courses have been instituted with considerable success. Quite apart from our serious doubts as to whether a course designed on these lines could achieve the kind of training needed, there would be other strong objections. The practical difficulties of arranging paid placements, providing for student supervision in them and keeping them vacant when they are not required, are daunting. We decided for all these reasons that we could not recommend 'sandwich' training.

8. We had also to consider whether it would meet the needs of the situation if a whole series of new specialized courses were recommended for work with the elderly, the physically handicapped, the mentally disordered, the socially handicapped[1] and other groups. We examined this question with great thoroughness (see paras. 17–22 below). Witnesses had said that usually people are attracted to residential work because of a strong interest in a particular group, whether it be children, adolescents, old people, the handicapped or others, and that they might expect to find all training courses narrowly focussed on their particular field. However we realized the proliferation and wastage that such a development of training schemes would entail and regarded such a solution as out of court, even if there were not very good reasons for its rejection on other counts.

9. We therefore looked closely at the arguments in favour of a common training for all forms of residential work and came to the unanimous conclusion that we should recommend a comprehensive course designed on these lines. It would occupy two years and would have a common core of subjects together with special options enabling the student to concentrate on one or more of his fields of interest (see paras. 23–33).

[1] There are a number of groups whom we have classed together as the 'socially handicapped' for want of a better term. We include in this group the mentally disordered and all those who for one reason or another are in need of residential care because they are unable to cope with ordinary life. This category includes mentally ill and mentally subnormal children and adults, delinquents, ex-prisoners, alcoholics, persons without a settled way of life and families who need help through residential care.

10. We were strengthened in our views by the evidence we had received. For instance, the Residential Child Care Association is convinced that training facilities, which are largely represented by the basic courses of a year in duration, are 'totally inadequate to meet the needs of the present service'. From other sources came evidence that the present basic course for work with children alone cannot be adequately carried out in one year.

11. Clearly the main object of any newly-designed course must be to give students a deeper understanding of the responsibilities and potentialities of residential care work: in short, that they may do the best possible job for the people in their care. The amount of ground to be covered in the proposed comprehensive course is necessarily extensive, given the broad scope of the syllabus and the need to provide sufficient well-integrated practical experience. To suggest anything less than a two-year course would therefore seem irresponsible; to suggest more would not be realistic. We make our recommendation knowing full well that there is a severe shortage of trained staff even in the child care field where training for residential work has been offered for twenty years, while in the other fields the provision has been limited. Nevertheless we are convinced that no shorter course would be adequate for what must ultimately be a new professional group within the social services.

12. While we recommend that the proposed comprehensive Two Year Course should be accepted as the normal preparation for those who wish to take up residential work as a career, we realize that it would not be practicable to suggest that in the present situation all staff and all new recruits, whatever their age or previous experience, should take a course of this kind. We therefore propose the establishment of one-year courses, with a minimum age limit, for work with the elderly, the physically handicapped and the socially handicapped to correspond with those already established in residential child care, although such courses will inevitably possess considerable limitations, as is apparent from paras. 37–40 below.

13. We further propose the stepping-up and co-ordination of in-service and staff development schemes, though these should not be regarded as an alternative to full-time training (paras. 45–49).

14. In addition, we look to the establishment of a considerable variety and number of Advanced Courses for all types of residential work (paras. 41–44). Some of these should be one year courses at post-graduate or post-certificate level and the contribution already made by the Advanced Courses at the Universities of Bristol and Newcastle rpovides most helpful precedent and experience. Others might be

short intensive courses for those undertaking wide or special responsibilities and would deal with particular aspects and new developments of the work.

15. We consider that all those in charge of Homes, their deputies and any others who carry any considerable responsibility for residents should have one or other type of full-time training. Other members of staff should have the opportunity of in-service training through a staff development programme in those cases where a formal course is considered inappropriate. It is most important that all staff should be brought into the programme of training or staff development at the appropriate point. One of the tasks of the staff with both training and experience will be to give guidance and support to inexperienced or partly trained colleagues and by this means the influence of a core of trained people will increasingly spread over the whole field.

16. As to existing training facilities, there is at present a one-year course for residential child care staff held in fifteen centres, which can be followed by a one-year Advanced Course (referred to above) after at least three years' experience. As the tables in Chapter 4 show, only 18 per cent of the staff in post in Children's Homes hold the residential Child Care Certificate or its equivalent, and 18 per cent have taken some other form of training; in Old People's Homes, 84 per cent of all staff have no qualifications and, for the most part those who are qualified have a general nursing qualification; only 2 per cent have a specific qualification in the residential care of old people, having taken the 14-week course for residential work with old people organized by the National Old People's Welfare Council. We pay tribute to this body which has pioneered this course and certain other short 'refresher' courses, but there is nothing of the standard considered by the Committee, or indeed by the National Old People's Welfare Council, to be anything like adequate. We also pay tribute to the Josephine Butler College which provides courses for those working with unmarried mothers. For those intending to work with socially handicapped people no training courses exist, although we recognize the value of the experiments which have been made with short courses by the National Association for Mental Health and one or two other bodies.

THE CASE FOR COMMON TRAINING FOR ALL TYPES OF RESIDENTIAL WORKS

17. Although a common training for the different fields of social work is becoming generally accepted, we did not feel able to assume that the same principles applied to the wide range of work in residen-

tial establishments. We therefore examined their relevance with great care. It became evident that there were many subjects which would necessarily have to be included in training for work with *any* residential group. Clearly all for whom this training is suggested would need to learn how to run a Home. All would need to study the development of human beings at all ages, since human life and needs cannot be considered in water-tight compartments. Indeed they would often have to deal with the families or relatives of residents whose age range and whose problems, quite apart from those of the residents themselves, would vary widely. All would need to understand as much as possible of group relationships and learn to use this knowledge. A further essential subject of study would be the structure of the social services, not only for its educational value but also because it shows how these develop and how provisions in a particular field of work relate to other groups and situations.

18. At first sight, when the two extremes—the care of children and the care of the elderly—are placed in juxtaposition, it might seem that the role of the residential worker is very different for the two groups, as indeed it is. For the one, he must be able to recognize and encourage growth processes in individual children and create an environment in which these may thrive; for the other, he may be dealing with adults who find it hard to accept their need for a supportive environment and where it is essential to have understanding of the physical and psychological implications of degenerative processes and terminal illness. But it must be remembered that, whether the aim is to provide a long term sheltered environment, temporary care and rehabilitation, a home that replaces the care a family would normally give, remedial work with disturbed children or adults or the care of elderly people with widely varying needs, so far as the residents are concerned they all make one basic demand on the residential worker. They all need understanding and help for themselves as individuals. It is the sustaining of personality with which the worker is concerned, and his task, though it will vary in method, is basically the same in purpose and intention for all ages and all groups.

19. The teaching in common of the basic elements relevant to all types of residential care must lead to a more economic deployment of lecturers, supervisors and training sources. The stimulation that comes from working alongside other students with a somewhat different approach and interest must be considerable and it cannot but encourage the students to think of themselves—and to be so regarded by others —as members of a social service of considerable significance.

20. The common training would also open up more varied career

prospects to students and facilitate change from one kind of residential work to another, after a short period of planned preparation. The extent to which in the future, if such a common training is established, there would be mobility and interchange within various areas of residential care cannot be gauged, but the possibility of transferring at some point to different but allied fields will underline the attractions of such a career. Some interchange of staff in post and the stimulation which comes from the pooling of ideas between workers with a variety of different approaches and responsibilities, cannot fail to be beneficial to residents and staff.

21.   Clearly the teaching given must fully meet the demands of the job. Those entering the field of child care, for instance, must be convinced that what they will be offered will be training of greater extent and depth than is possible in the existing courses. In the proposed course the emphasis would be placed fairly and squarely on training residential care workers, and on giving particular skills and knowledge in one or more areas of work. As we have said earlier, two years will be none too long to do justice to the common core of knowledge and its general and special application.

22.   The Committee has therefore, after very careful consideration, come to the unanimous conclusion that students wishing to undertake residential work of whatever kind should be trained together on common courses. The care of people in residential settings is a many-sided job of considerable complexity. A comprehensive, widely-based training course will do much to give staff the satisfaction of being equipped to do their work as effectively as possible and take their place as colleagues with nurses, social workers, teachers and others working to serve the widest needs of the community.

THE TWO-YEAR COURSE

23.   The Committee propose the establishment of a Two-year course to consist of a common basis and options to be selected by students in accordance with their special interests and that this shall be the normal method of entry into residential work. The purpose of such a course is to enable students to acquire the background, knowledge and practical skills of residential care on a general and comprehensive basis. It would lead to a growing self-awareness on the part of the student, and the cultivation of an ability to meet others, both residents and staff, with 'acceptance' in the residential situation, together with a particular appreciation of the needs of residents in one or more special fields. The course should provide a learning situation in which, at a number of

levels, experience is gained and understanding takes place, stimulated by tutors, lecturers and fellow students at a training centre, and by 'supervisors' and residents in a number of practical work placements. (By the 'supervisor' we mean the person who is primarily responsible for the student's learning whilst in a practical work placement. It may well be in larger establishments some of his responsibilities would be shared with other members of staff.) It would be essential to maintain close contact between tutors and supervisors, so as to integrate what is learnt at the centre with experience gained in residential settings.

24. Whilst there is less assembled information on which to base the teaching of residential care than, for example, in the related sphere of social work, published studies of life in residential communities are increasingly available. Studies by educational psychologists such as Susan Isaacs and Piaget, by social psychologists such as Moreno and others particularly concerned with life in residential settings—Aichhorn, Homer Lane, Wills, Lyward, Turner, T. and P. Morris and Townsend—have been augmented by more direct research, for example, in this country by Howard Jones, Derek Miller and Michael Craft. In the United States important contributions have been made by Bettelheim, Burmeister, Fenton, Konopka, Maier, Polsky, Rapaport and Redl to name but a few. United Nations publications increasingly carry reports of research work in residential settings. It is clear that more needs to be recorded of group work and group living in residential settings, especially by those in the work; however, a body of knowledge, some of it referred to above, some from studies published and unpublished and some from autobiography and novels, can provide a basis for the teaching of such a course as is proposed.

25. It is impossible to over-emphasize the importance of the role of the tutor in this kind of course. At the outset of such courses a difficulty will be the fact that, because the spheres of work have been separate in the past, few potential tutors will have had experience of more than one field, and teaching to be meaningful and appropriate will need to cull illustrations from different fields. To some extent this difficulty can be met by appointing to one course tutors whose experience has been in different fields, so that they can complement each other in this respect, but it should be made possible for tutors to gain experience at an early date in fields other than their own.

26. Certain basic subjects, as instanced in paragraph 17, would need to be covered by all students in the first year of the course envisaged. Students would also be encouraged to develop their own interests, so that later they would be enabled to do better work because they had more to give, and would have resources within themselves to match

up to the strains of residential life. In the second year, study of some of these basic subjects would continue but there would in addition be a focus on consideration of the special needs of certain particular groups, and the social services and residential communities provided for them.

27.　The particular fields of work which we consider warrant consideration as a separate option or special subjects are (A) children and young people; (B) the elderly; (C) the physically handicapped of all ages; and (D) the socially handicapped (with special reference to the mentally disordered and the socially maladjusted).

28.　Throughout their training, students will be prepared for living and working in a residential setting and their learning will need to be closely related to practical experience. It is therefore recommended that approximately half their time should be spent in residential placements where skilled guidance is available. Students should gain experience in a number of different residential settings and these would be arranged by the course tutors to meet the student's individual needs. In these settings students should not take the place of members of staff but would be supernumerary to the normal complement, working to a programme prepared for them by a supervisor in close association with the course tutor. This will be a time not merely for acquiring practical skill, but for integrating knowledge gained in lectures and tutorials with their practical experience and adjusting their approach to residential situations.

29.　One of the advantages of a training course designed in the way proposed is that a range of choice in subject matter and practical experience will be available. According to their particular interests students will be able to select one or more of the special four options mentioned above.

30.　In addition to the common content inherent in the course, there will be a considerable measure of common content between the special subjects and this should enable an additional number of lectures to be shared. It is not suggested that all the centres at which the two-year course might be given would offer all four special subjects, but rather that they would offer those which were appropriate to their situation and resources. The students would indicate their choice of special subjects at the commencement of the course, and if they desired to make a change, this should be possible at the end of the first year either at the same course centre, or if necessary by transfer to centres elsewhere.

31.　A suggested syllabus for the course is set out in Appendix C of this Report; it will be noted that practical work and work at the course centre are given equal significance; the exact balance struck between them, and the actual arrangements for practical work placements and time spent at the course centre, will vary with the different courses. Tutors will need to experiment in this; for such two-year courses there is not as yet any tried and established pattern of teaching and learning; the path is open and untrodden.

32. It is recommended that the minimum age of entry to this course should be 18, and we do not wish to suggest any upper age limit.

33. It is further recommended that a Certificate in Residential Care, which indicated the fields in which the student had specialized, be awarded by an appropriate national training body on the successful completion of such a course.

THE LOCATION OF THE COURSES

34. The Committee suggest that it is within the Colleges of Further Education that the courses will normally be established. In these, the students will be able to work alongside others in allied fields like social work with whom they may well study subjects of common interest. They will form part of an educational institution, with the advantage of common rooms and dining-rooms shared with students who are pursuing other subjects and disciplines, and the environment should prove stimulating and supportive.

35. A number of such colleges have established Departments of Social Studies and it is in these that the courses would normally be located. Some Residential Adult Education Colleges, University Extra-Mural Departments and Colleges of Education might also appropriately provide facilities for such courses. It is important that the students should feel an identity with an educational institution of some standing.

36. In the field of residential care, the provision of training courses has been pioneered by voluntary organizations and it is hoped that they, too, would consider in the new situation the provision of the wider training envisaged. Whilst we would recommend that such training should be given in association with an educational establishment they might well contribute with their exceptional experience to the teaching of special subjects within the general pattern of training.

A ONE-YEAR COURSE

37. It is hoped to attract many men and women to residential work in their middle years. Some may want to change their job after 20 or 30 years; others, women in particular, will have left the work in which

they were engaged before marriage to bring up their families and when they are no longer tied by them, might well turn to residential work. They should find it a satisfying and worthwhile job to which they could bring their experiences of parenthood and housekeeping as well as a mature approach to life.

38.   For those aged 35 and over we recognize that a one-year course may be realistic and appropriate. This will be particularly useful for those who have had some years of residential or other relevant experience. Courses are already provided for those working with children and young people, the minimum age of entry for which is 18 years. We hope, however, that these will develop into two-year courses as we recommend. As these become established, the one-year courses which remain should be confined to mature students over 35. For older students who wish to work with the other groups, we recommend that additional specialized one-year courses be established. Teaching on the basic 'common' subjects would have to be reduced, but it would still be important to maintain a balance between class-room and practical teaching. The courses should be based on an appropriate educational institution where Two-year courses are being held.

39.   We recommend, in order that there should be one Certificate (apart from any advanced qualification), easily recognizable in the whole field of residential care, that this Certificate should be awarded for both the two-year and the one-year courses, indicating that the student has taken a qualification in the field of residential care. The Certificate should state the special field or fields of study and the length of the particular course taken. To this extent, the courses will have parity of esteem. However, some students over the age of 35 may well prefer to take a two-year course because of the greater understanding that follows a longer period of study and of the wider employment opportunities that should result from such a course.

40.   We recommend that the provision of the proposed One-year courses should be for five years in the first instance. These should be kept under review by the national body responsible for training, to assess how they work in relation to the Two-year Course, whether any alteration needs to be made in such special provision, or indeed whether it should be continued.

ADVANCED COURSES IN RESIDENTIAL CARE

41.   Courses at a more advanced level, designed for mature, experienced and qualified staff should be developed to meet a number of different needs. These would cater for those wanting to develop their

own skills in group processes and therapeutic influences, and those who are preparing to undertake considerable additional responsibility for residents and staff and for the training of staff.

42. It might well be that the present two Advanced courses—each lasting for a full academic year and already taking students from a range of residential settings—might be prepared to consider accepting students from even more varied backgrounds. It is hoped too, that other Universities would consider the provision of such courses on a generic basis, and take students from the whole field of residential work. Entry to these courses would be primarily intended for those who have taken the two-year course and have had considerable experience, but we recommend that other entrants coming from related fields should be considered in exceptional circumstances without this particular qualification, if they have appropriate and relevant training and experience. It is believed that a limited number of graduates and some members of allied professions such as nurses, social workers and teachers may wish to take up residential work. They could make a valuable contribution, though few of them would be qualified to undertake responsible positions in this field without some further training. Advice on the appropriate course should be available from the national body responsible for training.

43. When University Departments include in their Diploma of Education Courses teaching and practical work in residential settings and in their Applied Social Studies Courses the opportunity for postgraduate and post-certificate students to specialize in group work, there should be a welcome entry into residential work of people with new skills and experience in both the residential and non-residential fields.

44. Appropriate academic awards should be issued on the successful completion of Advanced Courses lasting a year or more.

IN-SERVICE TRAINING AND STAFF DEVELOPMENT

45. Proper care for clients in residence requires, in addition to the institution of recognized training courses, the establishment of in-service training and staff development projects. Provision has to be made in this context for staff of a wide range of ability and of varying ages on entry. Differing attitudes towards residential work will need to be taken into consideration and the degree of responsibility which staff are likely to assume. It is not envisaged that all will take the

same type of training, but, because of the importance of any work with people in a residential setting, all should have at least some form of introductory training in residential care.

46. We believe that every entrant into the work should have an introductory course. This would be planned to meet differing needs and capabilities. For students about to take a full-time training it would involve preliminary reading and some guidance by a senior member of staff. Introductory courses for staff for whom a full-time training is considered inappropriate because of home ties, restricted responsibilities, personal limitations or very late entry into the work, should be integrated with an in-service training scheme. Such training might be given in a variety of ways, such as individual study, or attendance at a study group arranged within the establishment, conducted by a member of the residential staff or a visiting tutor, or both; or it might be on a day-release basis and held in a convenient centre. It would involve selected reading, and would be related to the needs and capabilities of the individual staff member.

47. Staff who have completed a training course leading to a certificate should have opportunities for continued study; these would be of particular significance on promotion, on transfer from one area of residential work to another, and for those wishing to acquire management skills for large units or groups of Homes. From this group will come most of those who would later be suitable for an advanced course and those who show exceptional ability should be encouraged to obtain the higher qualification. Seminars and short refresher courses with different emphases, opportunities for staff discussion and consultation and conferences organized by professional associations, all have their place in a staff development programme.

48. Residential institutions will inevitably have a significant part to play in relation to the whole training programme. In laying down the functions of senior staff, their role in training will need to be recognized and the supervision of students and the carrying through of staff development programmes regarded as an integral and important part of their responsibilities.

49. It may be that it will prove advisable to group institutions for training purposes and to designate some staff primarily for this task. In addition to the contribution of residential staff, local authorities may decide to appoint non-resident staff to act as tutors in charge of a training programme designed to meet the needs of a very broad band of staff. Some voluntary bodies may continue to make similar appointments. Some course centres too may see a need to appoint peripatetic tutors and advisers. Thus a comprehensive staff development pro-

gramme may evolve to operate in residential settings, course centres and elsewhere. Staff development should be seen as a continuous and never-ending process.

JUNIOR OR 'PRELIMINARY' TRAINING

50. In Chapter 7 when discussing recruitment it was suggested that young women interested in work with people might be employed under suitable conditions to help care for adults or children in residence, to the benefit of all concerned. While these conditions included supervision in which they would be helped to learn from their experience, it was not envisaged that this would in any sense be systematic training. It was, however, recognized that some girls who have reached a good level of education often want to undertake training before they enter employment and may turn to quite other occupations if they cannot start any course until the age of eighteen. It is partly this consideration which has led in the field of child care to the younger age for a training for nursery nurses, to the cadet schemes of some of the large voluntary organizations and, more recently, to two-year 'preliminary' or 'junior' courses for residential work with children based upon Colleges of Further Education.

51. Training for girls of this age seems to us to fall more properly under the auspices of educational establishments than of particular voluntary organizations or local authorities in terms of their own service. However disinterestedly they are designed, cadet schemes suggest future commitment, and the training given by a particular service for its own ends tends to become ingrown. Moreover, courses designed wholly for residential work, particularly if they are related only to the care of one age group, such as children of under five, are likely to prevent a healthy variety of experience and a broadening of outlook which should be particularly encouraged at this age. If young people are offered a two-year training solely for residential work before the age of eighteen, it would be unreasonable to expect them to undertake a further two years when they are more mature, and it is very unlikely that more than a few would be willing to do so.

52. A good case, however, can be made for providing full- or part-time courses in Colleges of Further Education or at centres provided by voluntary organizations, designed as continued education both general and vocational, and as an introduction to social service in its broader sense. Such courses might provide classes in home-making and house-keeping and also in such subjects as the social services, government, health and leisure time activities and illustrated by visits when-

ever possible. Experience could be gained not only in residential institutions for adults and children and for subnormal children, but also in such services as maternity and child welfare, in old people's clubs and Homes, nursery schools and play centres. They could provide a useful introduction for some young people who would later take up residential work or go into other branches of the social services, as well as ensuring that they would be better fitted to be parents and better educated as citizens. If the course has been satisfactorily completed, the Colleges will no doubt give the students whatever recognition they think appropriate, though this should not appear to be in any sense a 'qualification'.

53. As and when the school leaving age is raised to 16 years, the last year might, with advantage, be spent by a number of both boys and girls in similar fashion; there would be a real place here for introducing them to residential care as well as to other social services, and to tap the very considerable interest in personal service that exists in young people but which cannot always find expression.

NURSES

54. At present a number of Homes for elderly people, for mothers and babies, for the physically handicapped, and for very young children, have as their matron or head a trained nurse. This has been the result of the lack of recognized training for residential work in these fields and the anxiety of the employing bodies to ensure that there is some trained person on the staff even if the training has not been wholly relevant. This trend has been followed in a number of other establishments with less justification.

55. We were impressed by the evidence from the Royal College of Nursing which pointed out that trained nurses were too scarce to be employed in residential Homes except where a great deal of nursing skill was required. 'Nurses,' they said, 'should not be used to look after healthy people.'

56. With the development of a comprehensive training scheme, it may well be argued that it would as a rule be wasteful and improper to appoint nurses to such positions. Their professional service as nurses might from time to time be needed in a number of Homes, and they could visit as required daily or nightly, but it would seem sensible to relieve them of other duties and so free them to apply their nursing skills, fully without the encumbrance of administrative responsibilities. This does not mean that with an appropriate qualification in residential care they would not be cordially welcomed in residential posts, but it

would seem wrong to staff Homes at the expense of hospitals and other places needing trained nurses.

57. There is, however, a further consideration. There are some Homes, such as those for handicapped babies and for infirm elderly persons requiring constant attention, where the presence of a nurse on the staff indicates the constant availability of proper medical and nursing care. This would be a reassuring factor for these elderly residents and their families, and a safeguard for those responsible for the care of such young children. It is not envisaged that such an arrangement in the comparatively small number of Homes concerned 'affects the general validity of the training programme already outlined.

58. In general, we think of the nurse as coming into Homes to give nursing care, supplementing the skills of the residential care workers in this respect. In a few cases they might be the administrative heads or deputy heads of establishments, and if so, they would still need some training in residential work. Whether this should be a Two-year or a One-year course, or one of the courses provided under the heading of staff development in the form of an orientation course, would need to be considered in each individual case and in relation to past training and experience.

A NATIONAL TRAINING BODY

59. Our proposals for a comprehensive training scheme inevitably led us to consider how to ensure the provision of courses and the adoption of nationally recognized standards of work in the field of residential care.

60. The training programme of the Central Training Council in child care has provided the only experience of courses leading to a national qualification for residential work and this exclusively for work with children and young people. This council, set up in 1947 to deal with the whole child care field, has as one of its responsibilities training courses for residential staff. It advises on syllabus, promotes new courses, awards a 'Certificate in the Residential Care of Children' to successful students, and is responsible for the maintenance of training standards. In 18 years, about 3,000 students have qualified for its Certificate. The Advisory Council for Probation and After-Care also has responsibilities in the residential field, but for this purpose it has called upon the service of the Home Office as advised by the Central Training Council in Child Care. We are fully satisfied that, in order to achieve our recommendations over the whole field of residential care, a new training body is needed with comparable but broader responsibilities, and able

to deal with all the groups for whom residential care is provided, i.e. people in all age groups whatever their needs or handicaps or social inadequacies.

61. Such a body would clearly need to look for help and guidance to those already in the field of residential care or allied fields, but it would also have to break much new ground and seek the help of other disciplines. It would promote courses and advise on their planning and content, the selection of students, the establishment and maintenance of standards in training and would assist in the setting up of in-service training and staff development courses. It would award a qualification —most probably a Certificate in Residential Care.

62. This body would have an extremely important additional function, namely to concern itself with promoting and assisting with enquiries and research in this whole field. The Committee has been very conscious of the many areas in which research is needed in relation to residential care, including size and planning of buildings, the interpretation of the needs of residents, and the differing reactions of residents and staff to such provision.

63. The Committee is anxious that its proposals should incidentally encourage a closer working relationship between those engaged in residential care work on the one hand and field social workers on the others. They would therefore regard it as unfortunate if a new training body were established which was only concerned with the residential field. It is common knowledge that the existence of three national Training Councils concerned with social work in the fields of child care, probation and health and welfare is a source of embarrassment and overlapping to those responsible for the development of those services and the Committee trust that the Government will take steps to bring them together. In this event they would hope that a Council for Training in Social Work and Residential Care would be constituted which would maintain balanced interests in these two complementary fields. It would thus be able to foster the common concern of both types of worker, encourage greater interchange of experience during and after training, and economize in the use of tutors and other teaching staff. Such a Council should be set up as an independent body, and supported from public funds. It would need a Director of high qualifications and experience and a professional staff of appropriate size.

64. The Committee, however, is aware that in order to implement this recommendation fully, legislation would be required and this in turn takes time. We therefore recommend, as a temporary and immediate expedient, that the three existing Councils should each designate

some of their members to form an interim Council for Training in Residential Care, charged with the promotion of pilot courses of the type which we have proposed. This interim Council would have no doubt to be responsible to, and derive its authority from, each of the three Councils, and in view of the experimental nature of some of its work the support and interest of voluntary trusts should be enlisted. However, it is to be hoped that the life of such a liaison Council would be quite brief and not exceed two years, which could be used largely as a demonstration period.

65. The Committee are reluctant to contemplate a situation in which three Training Councils continue to exist independently. However, in the event of this remaining Government policy, they would then favour and indeed wish to press for the immediate setting up of a fourth Council—a Council for Training in Residential Care, concerned with training in this field. They consider it imperative that there should be a body responsible for developing training on the lines proposed, in order that workers in this whole field should have the support they deserve for such demanding work and the sense of following a career that is in the national interest and is seen to be one that demands sound training and offers fitting rewards.

FINANCE

66. The national training body, or the Committee which may stand in for it as a temporary expedient, will need funds for its own staff and administration, for giving grants to courses in special circumstances as, for example, those provided by voluntary bodies, and for general supportive work, such as preparing tutors and those who teach students when they are learning to apply in a residential setting what they have studied in the classroom. We recommend that these funds should be provided by the Exchequer.

67. It is presumed that students training for residential work will be eligible for local education authority grants or grants from the Scottish Education Department as the case may be. It has been put to us in evidence that in the past students have been discouraged from taking training by inadequate grants—however provided—and in particular that older students with families (unless they have been able to secure secondment on salary from a residential post) have been particularly hard hit or altogether deterred. Grants should be adequate; in addition, expenses that are necessarily incurred by students in the course of their training should be paid promptly and in full.

68. Secondment of staff for training on full salary can prove expensive

for the individual authority; because of great differences between authorities in their policy about secondment, the more liberal may in practice subsidize other authorities, for trained staff may leave after meeting their minimum obligations in order to move to more responsible positions elsewhere. There seems to be no answer to this dilemma except some form of pooling expenses between local authorities for staff seconded for training, and we recommend that some appropriate form of pooling should be considered for this purpose, as is already done in some fields.

69. Financial support for students of courses in residential care should be available whether the courses are established by local authority Colleges of Further Education, by Extra-Mural Departments of Universities, by Adult Colleges or big voluntary organizations, provided the courses are recognized by the central training body.

70. We recommend that the establishment of courses should normally be the financial responsibility of local education authorities, as are the courses leading to the Certificate in Social Work; we are confident that an adequate number of authorities will be willing to promote this new form of training.

71. An advanced course, lasting one year, will it is hoped be established within universities as are the two courses already in existence. It is hoped that University authorities will appreciate the high social priorities involved and will encourage the setting up of the relatively few advanced courses that are likely to be necessary.

72. We hope that charitable trusts would be prepared to make a significant contribution to the development of training. They might for example make it possible for certain residential homes to become special 'training centres' for students' practical training; or provide intending tutors or supervisors with opportunities to prepare themselves for their work and responsibilities; or promote experiment and research into training for residential care including in-service training and staff development.

73. However, training for a large number of people, and for some of these for a relatively long period, must involve the expenditure of a considerable amount of public money. The burden of this Report is the need for staff to be trained for residential care and in our view the case for the expenditure involved is incontravertible.

RECOGNITION OF EXPERIENCE

74. The main recommendation in this chapter is the establishment of a considerable number of courses of both common and special content

which shall last for two years. These courses will be supplemented by one-year specialized courses, proposed for a limited period at this juncture, and by an intensive in-service and staff development programme. Training will further be developed by Advanced Courses set up to meet particular needs. These courses should not be confined to future recruits only; secondment of present staff should make it possible for many of them to take advantage of these provisions.

75. There will be a considerable number, however, for whom, apart from in-service training and staff development, little provision can be made. These are experienced older people for many of whom there have existed totally insufficient facilities for training in the past, and, whilst they will welcome the setting up of a comprehensive training scheme, they will be distressed that they are unable to take advantage of it. It will not be easy to devise a formula for recognition of their experience, but the Home Office is proceeding so to do for those that come within its purview and we would urge the other Government Departments to proceed along the same lines for staff for whom they have a comparable responsibility. We are not able to advise how and on what terms this should be done and the operative dates and the definition of relevant experience will not be easy to decide. But we would encourage the training body, if so requested, to co-operate in such a scheme, although we do not recommend that they take the responsibility of implementing it.

RECOMMENDATIONS

1. Training for all forms of residential care is essential. (Paras 1–5.)

2. The accepted pattern of training for those who wish to take up residential work as a career should be a two-year course providing a common content of study for all students, with special sections enabling the student to concentrate on his main fields of interest. (Paras 8–11, 17–33 and Appendix C.)

3. For some older and experienced students, a one-year course of a specialized nature should be set up, in the first instance for an experimental period of 5 years. (Paras 12, 37–40.)

4. Two-year and one-year courses should be based on a recognized educational institution, normally a College of Further Education. (Paras 34–36.)

5. Students who successfully complete a two-year course or a one-year course should receive a nationally recognized Certificate in Residential Care. (Paras 33, 39, 61.)

6. There should be a total training programme which would also provide for Advanced Courses at University level, and schemes for in-service and staff development. Appropriate training of some type should be available to all staff having the care of residents. (Paras 13–15, 41–49.)

7. Junior or preliminary courses should be provided for young people on leaving school. (Paras 50–53.)

8. A national training body should be established to foster training developments, set standards and encourage research. Preferably this should be an additional responsibility of the three existing statutory Training Councils when and if these are combined. (Paras 59–63.)

9. To ensure immediate progress in setting up the proposed courses, an Interim Council should be set up by the three existing Councils. (Paras 64–65.)

10. The cost of financing training should be met from public funds —from the Exchequer to finance the national training body and from local education grants to finance students. A pooling arrangement to finance staff seconded for training should be established. (Paras 66–73.)

11. There should be a scheme which provides for the recognition of experience. (Paras 74–75.)

SUMMARY OF PROPOSALS FOR TRAINING COURSES

76. The following is a very brief summary of our recommendations on training courses. It is highly condensed for the sake of clarity, and must be read in conjunction with the fuller description of the courses in Chapter 8 and Appendix C.

Course	Students	Location
Two Year Course		
First year—common curriculum	Normally for new recruits aged 18 and over; younger staff in post	Colleges of Further Education and other training centres
Second Year—one or two options:		
(a) Children		
(b) Elderly		
(c) Physically handicapped		
(d) Socially handicapped		

Course	Students	Location
One Year Course In one specialization only: (*a*) Children (*b*) Elderly (*c*) Physically handicapped (*d*) Socially handicapped	For new recruits aged 35 and over; older staff in post	Colleges of Further Education and other training centres
Advanced Courses Common curriculum	Normally staff with basic training (one or two year course) and considerable experience	Universities
Staff development	In-service training for staff without other training and new entrants who cannot take full-time training because of home ties, etc. Refresher courses for all staff	On the job training with part-time teaching through Colleges of Further Education, residential colleges, etc.

All training to include integrated theory and practice.

General Introductory Courses		
Not confined to residential work. Full or part-time	Potential recruits aged 16–18	Colleges of Further Education

9

COMMUNITY AND COMMITTEE

1. Throughout this Report we have constantly emphasized the importance we attach to the forging of close links between a residential Home and the neighbourhood near to it. Fortunately the large majority of Homes are situated sufficiently near to residential areas for this to be practicable; but it does not inevitably come about of itself without the efforts of those concerned. Yet it is worth considerable effort, for both residents and staff suffer if their lives are cut off from those amongst whom they live.

2. How can members of a Committee responsible for a Home, either individually or collectively, support the staff and ensure satisfactory standards of care? To judge by the replies we have received to these questions, Committees are as various as the establishments they manage, and so are the ways in which they are recruited, their degrees of expertise, and their sensitiveness to the task. These are some examples of adverse comments which have come to us.

'They assume they can walk in at any hour of the day or night without so much as knocking.' 'I am not even invited to sit down when called to the Committee Room for discussion.' 'Some members only know the name of the headmaster, and have never spoken to a single boy.' 'One of the most difficult things is to get rid of a voluntary Committee.' 'They are so busy raising money that they have no time to think about the work itself.'

3. But there is no doubt that, under a wide variety of patterns of management, the staff of many Homes and schools have extremely good relations with the Committee which is ultimately responsible and we have tried to analyse the elements which make for good relationships and efficient management.

4. It would be tempting simply to differentiate Homes and schools under the direct management of Local Authorities from those administered by voluntary societies. But we found both Local Authority

and voluntary management (taking the large voluntary bodies) faced the same problems and dealt with them in a wide variety of ways. Sometimes Homes were managed from afar by national or regional bodies; sometimes by sub-committees of those bodies; sometimes without any committee but under the general oversight of a chief officer. Only in the case of approved and special schools was the pattern more uniform under regulations of management laid down by the appropriate Central Government departments: in both cases a Board of Management is directly responsible for the school.

5. One group of Homes we had to distinguish. These were those provided by small voluntary organizations which in many cases were responsible for a single Home. They had generally been established by a small group of people who had mobilized the necessary funds to meet an urgent local need. Sometimes the initial impetus of planning and fund-raising was not matched with knowedge of contemporary social work or management, and we felt much concerned for the staff of these Homes where there are no consultants to turn to and which seemed to us to be out of touch with the main stream of development in the social services. It is not easy for those who have put much thought, time and energy into creating a Home to realize that they may not be the right persons to play a big part in the administration once it is in being.

6. Whatever the pattern and however remote the control over the Home, there are certain collective functions that some body of people outside the Home itself must ultimately exercise.

7. Of these, the most obvious is the provision and control of money. Whether these funds on which the Home depends are provided by the Local Authority, are raised by charging fees or come from voluntary contributions, it is necessary that care should be taken of how the money is spent, and the managing body must determine the order of priorities. The head of a Home may have some discretion in the laying out of the funds; the practice and degree of discretion vary. But it is the managing Committee which must allocate the funds within broad categories of expenditure and ensure that a reasonable amount of economy and good sense is shown in the actual spending.

8. Once a Home is in being, the Committee may feel that extra funds for special amenities might be raised by 'open days', coffee mornings and the like at the Home, and we came across instances of such functions, not all of them desirable and not all of them confined to voluntary Homes. Moral pressure was sometimes exerted by the Committee on the staff to add the job of fund-raising to their duties. We heard of open days for fund-raising and other purposes which, particularly in

old people's homes, seemed to ignore the residents as though they had no part in such functions. On the other hand, many heads of Homes shared with their Committees the conception of using an open day to bring the wider community to the Home, to give the residents an opportunity to act on such occasions as hosts in their own Homes, and to consult the residents as to the spending of any funds which resulted. In statutory and voluntary Homes alike this seemed to us commendable, so long as the Committee did not see it as a main focus of its endeavours.

9. The Committee is responsible for the employment of staff, their proper remuneration and their conditions of service. Whether it devolves this work to its Chairman, to sub-committees, designated members or chief officers, it is the Committee which must assume collective responsibility for the engagement and dismissal of staff. In most cases responsibility, at least for the appointment of heads of homes, is exercised by the Committee itself and we do not consider that heads should be allowed to appoint their own deputies, although they should be consulted fully about these appointments. On the other hand, particularly in some Local Authority contexts, we feel it an infringement of the responsibility of senior paid officers, and a waste of public time and money, that Committees should themselves wish to appoint the most junior members of staff. Enough has been said in other chapters about the proper remuneration and living conditions of staff to make it clear that we feel a Committee has a collective responsibility to assure itself that pay and conditions conform to nationally acceptable standards.

10. Out of the Committee's responsibility for the appointment of staff arises its further responsibility for supporting the staff when difficulties arise. Where chief officers acting on the Committee's behalf are responsible for staffing they too have a right to look to the Committee for support in difficult situations, and the Committee must be careful not to undermine their authority by interfering in matters affecting the staff of the Home without first consulting them.

11. This assumes that the Committee collectively establishes a working relationship with heads and other senior officers of Homes, inviting them to attend relevant meetings and taking their point of view on matters over which the Committee must take responsibility. Whether it is the appointment of staff or a determination of priorities of expenditure, consultation with staff is an essential for harmonious development.

12. Most important of all is the Committee's collective responsibility for the comfort and well-being of the residents. Sometimes this will

mean persuading the staff to alter their attitude in certain aspects of the running of the Home; the involvement of residents in simple tasks in the running of old people's Homes, even though the staff may not welcome it, was an example frequently quoted to us. Sometimes there may be complaints from residents about their conditions or their relations with the staff. The Committee must collectively put itself in a position to deal with complaints whether from the staff or the residents fairly and dispassionately. What is more, they must expect such difficulties, for residential communities, whatever the type of resident, always produce them.

13. Complaints do not always arise inside a Home. Sometimes they come from relatives and friends. It is the price that has sometimes to be paid for encouraging close links between residents and their families, in itself highly desirable; but not all relatives and friends are kind and considerate, and some of them may make it more, rather than less, difficult for residents to settle down. Parents of children in Homes and special schools may unconsciously grudge the independence and security their children gain in such settings; boy friends of unmarried mothers may be truculent and brash; fathers of homeless families, resentful.

14. We have referred several times during this report to the lack of knowledge and understanding on the part of the general public about what goes on in residential establishments and it is when crisis occurs that this is most likely to lead to uninformed strictures and criticism of those in charge. The other half of the duty to maintain standards and to protect the interests of the residents is that of standing as buffer between the staff and their critics. Criticisms and allegations must always be investigated; but if the Committee has already established feelings of friendly co-operation with the staff, such investigations will be accepted in the confidence and trust that the judgments will be fair and objective. The Committee may have to deal with complaints from senior staff about their juniors or from juniors about their seniors. Their role is to provide disinterested concern, unbiased judgment and a sense of perspective brought into the Home from the wider world outside.

15. So far we have attempted to describe what we see as the Committee's collective responsibility. But Committees consist of people, and we think it important to define the responsibility of individual committee members. In whatever setting they serve, Committee members are volunteers, elected or selected to participate in the collective function of management. They in themselves represent the wider community's interest in the well-being of the residents and staff.

16. Many of our witnesses and those we visited in their own establish-

ments spoke to us of the immense support they gained from helpful members of their Committees. In some cases it was the knowledge that there was always available some understanding listener to whom they could go with problems that seemed at the moment insoluble. In others it was the sense that the Home was not isolated but that there were people coming in to the Home who could gradually build up a relationship of friendliness and concern with both the residents and the members of staff.

17.   But the role of the individual Committee member is more subtle than this, for he has no standing in a Home unless he is designated by the Committee to fulfil a specific function. He must draw a careful line between demonstrating the interests of the community and throwing his weight about as a member of a Committee. He should not, for example, go as of right to visit the Home at all times and expect the staff or residents, whose home it is, to welcome him by virtue of his Committee membership.

18.   He has a duty to attend meetings regularly and he has a duty to acquaint himself with the professional roles of different members of staff and to respect the ethics of the professions they represent. He may require to know something of the background of the residents, but he must respect the confidentiality of information discussed in Committee, and should be careful not to demand as of right to be given information about individuals which he would not be given in full Committee.

19.   The duties and responsibilities we have outlined are so important and call for so much knowledge and tact that in an ideal situation we would wish Committee members to be appointed with as much care as members of the staff. Unfortunately this is by no means the situation. Very often members of Committees are appointed who have only a slight interest in the Homes they are called upon to manage, and once on the Committee, they are liable to stay there.

20.   Too often, Committees fail to establish a rota system by which some at least of their members change every year. The self-perpetuating Committee is found far too often. Here Local Authorities have an advantage, for the fortunes of election normally ensure some change in Committee membership. The unchanging Committees are a particular feature of the small voluntary bodies to which we have already referred.

21.   We have spoken of the Committee as representing the interest of the community in the welfare of the Home but there are other members of the community who should share in this. Happily there are many groups of well wishers in the community linked with voluntary bodies who bring the concern of their own organization into particular Homes.

The nursing auxiliaries of the Red Cross, the trolley shops of the W.V.S. and the friendly groups of the National Federation of Women's Institutes are examples. Other homes have organized groups of 'friends of the Home' undertaking stand-in jobs for the staff, providing parties and outings for residents, coming in to befriend residents who have no families. Many more people are ready to offer individual friendly and imaginative help—if only they know that this help is needed and appreciated.

22. The variety of opportunity and the wealth of goodwill is in fact so great that we are glad to find that a Committee of enquiry has now been established jointly by the National Council of Social Service and the National Institute for Social Work Training to examine the role of volunteers, their relationship to professional workers and the need for training or preparation.

23. Despite all this, it is clear to us that much requires to be done to improve the reserve of volunteers for Committee work and to enhance the status of their responsibilities. We believe that the net should be cast much more widely than at present—for example by making the need known to those in schools, industry, commerce, farming, and the various professional bodies which might offer people with specially needed expertise. We hope that some steps might be taken to free men and women in professional employment to give some part of their working time to the task of management. The skills for which it calls are not to be found exclusively in retired people and in the diminishing band of housewives with leisure time.

24. Once recruited we believe there is scope for new members to go to introductory courses where some of the ideas set out in this chapter might be explored. We know that the National Old People's Welfare Council has some experience in this direction, and the response they have received argues much good will on the part of Committee members. And why not, when Marriage Guidance Counsellors and Magistrates have shown themselves ready to train for their different responsibilities?

25. But this is not enough. We would welcome the expansion of the practice of some Local Authorities and voluntary bodies for members to hear direct from senior and junior members of staff at organized gatherings of the progress of their work and the particular difficulties they face. Conferences which members can attend with their officers are valuable, but there is also a need for separate meetings for Committee members.

26. The need to help Committee members in their responsibilities is clear. The opportunity to fill this gap and to see its importance for the

better management of Homes and schools means experiment and a willingness on the part of individuals and authorities alike to make it possible.

RECOMMENDATIONS

1.   Care should be taken to recruit members of Committees from as wide a section of the community as possible (Paras 19–20, 23).

2.   Care should be taken to appoint those who will undertake their duties seriously and be willing to prepare themselves for those duties (Paras 8–18).

3.   Experiments should be made in providing courses of preparation for Committee members (Paras 24–25).

4.   Encouragement should be given to establishing connecting links between the community and the Home (Paras 21–22).

10

CONCLUSION

1. The greater part of this Report is concerned with discussions of the present situation, the problems to be faced and the likely developments in the future for which provision must be made. It is not possible to summarize these discussions without distorting the argument and changing the emphasis. In many chapters, however, we make specific recommendations and these will be found at the end of the chapter to which they relate.

2. But whilst it is not possible to summarize the arguments, our discussions have raised a number of issues with regard to the staffing of residential Homes which are so important that we believe it is of value to draw special attention to them.

(i) For many reasons that have been set out in detail, the skills needed by the staffs are increasingly complex but unhappily the public remains ignorant of this fact and does not fully appreciate the nature of the work to be done.

(ii) There is a very great variation in the accommodation provided for members of staff who are resident in Homes and in the other conditions of employment. Some are admirable but there are too many instances in which they are far from attractive.

(iii) The lack of any clear career structure acts as a disincentive to many able and suitable people—especially young people—who would otherwise enter this field of employment. And many who are initially attracted do not remain in it.

(iv) We have made many recommendations which we believe would go far to deal with these difficulties but there is one group of recommendations which we believe to be supremely important—this is concerned with Training. We do not believe that training is a universal cure for all the problems to which we call attention; but we are quite certain that it is an essential element in any constructive plan for coping with them. This kind of skilled work cannot be done properly without adequate training, and incidentally good training also promotes recruitment and helps to make possible a reasonable career structure.

(v) The changes that have taken place in marriage rates in the pattern of family building have brought about profound alterations in the familiar field of recruitment for this occupation. The number of single women available for employment is rapidly decreasing. In the past this has been the main section of the community from which residential Homes have drawn their staffs and many Homes are still dependent on single women who are now approaching the age of retirement. There are not enough to replace them. This is a problem which faces many other occupations and those responsible for residential Homes will be forced to realize that they will be increasingly in competition for a constantly decreasing group of women. This involves a fundamental re-thinking of staffing structure.

RESEARCH

3. We cannot claim that we have considered every possible line of enquiry in this Report. We tried to collect information by means of our census and we have collected much evidence and many ideas from those working in this field. But the longer that the Committee worked the more aware we became of whole areas of ignorance. Some of these present such wide gaps in knowledge that we urge further study. We suggest here some of the topics which demand research:

(i) Almost nothing is known about the feelings of, for example, old people with regard to those who care for them. Do the majority like a small, cosy home or a large one with greater variety? What do they like to do? Do they feel insecure if the matron lives out? Or do they readily accept this?

The answer to questions such as these obviously affects the number and kind of staff needed but, at present, there has been so little Consumer Research that no valid answer can be given. Many experiments are being made in supplying different kinds of Homes—or sheltered housing—all over the country; but the experience gained in these experiments is not recorded and information that could be available is lost to an authority or organization which is planning new provision.

(ii) There are many plans to build a large number of hostels for the mentally ill but we are aware of no research to find out whether life in such a hostel is the best way of providing for those who need care. Nor do we know what staff should be employed.

(iii) We similarly need more knowledge of the value of very small children's Homes in relation to larger ones.

(iv) We know that on an average about a third of the staff in a children's Home both small and large leave every year but we do not know why. As continuity is particularly important for children we should find out why therei s such a rapid turnover, and how it might be reduced. The Social Survey study for the Home Office to which reference has been made in Chapter 1 is one of the few pieces of evidence on this matter.

(v) We need considerably more knowledge of the actual work to be done in a Home and the possible changes in equipment that might reduce the number of staff needed or reduce the strain on them. Specific studies of Homes would provide material of value to those who are planning new ones or converting old ones.

(vi) The problems of the children of the staff and their relations with the people in care require further study.

(vii) We do not know enough of the way in which a group of people living and working together in a Home develop into a community. Yet this is of great importance in deciding the kind of person who is likely to work happily with others as well as with the residents and so in influencing both recruitment and training.

(viii) It is generally accepted that it is important for members of staff to establish good relationships with the families and friends of those for whom they are caring as well as with other professional people with whom they have to co-operate. But we do not know how this good relationship and co-operation are brought about nor how it can best be fostered, although we realize it is done with considerable success by some staff.

(ix) We have devised certain training programmes that we believe will do much to improve the situation but there is need for constant validation. It is essential to be eternally vigilant to ensure that the training provided actually achieves what it sets out to do.

FINANCIAL IMPLICATIONS

4. We realize that the establishment of training courses, improved accommodation, shorter hours of work and the other changes in staff conditions which we have recommended will cost money. But unless this money is spent there is no hope of any significant improvement in the numbers and quality of the staff who enter and remain in residential work; and unless there is significant improvement in these respects it is not possible to provide the amount and quality of care that is needed. The happiness and welfare of the hundreds of thousands

who must be cared for in residential Homes depend on our willingness to spend this money. We do not consider the extra costs excessive in relation to the amount of human happiness involved.

APPENDIX A

LIST OF WITNESSES

The following submitted evidence to the Committee. Those marked with an asterisk submitted written evidence only. Those marked with a dagger, oral evidence only. The rest gave us both written and oral evidence.

Association of Charity Officers
Association of Children's Officers
Association of Directors of Welfare Services
Association of Hospital and Welfare Administrators
Association for Special Education
*Association of Workers for Maladjusted Children
*Association of Workers with Maladjusted Children, Scotland
†Mr C. J. Beedell
†Miss E. Bremer
*British Deaf and Dumb Association
British Red Cross Society
Church Army
*Church of England Council for Social Work
County Welfare Officers' Society
Mr and Mrs E. C. Crompton
Department of Education and Science
Dr Barnardo's Homes
*Elizabeth Fry Home, York
Guild of Catholic Professional Social Workers
Ministry of Health
Dr Robin Higgins
Home Office
Howard League for Penal Reform
*Mr R. E. Hughes
Institute of Social Welfare
Institutional Management Association
Jewish Welfare Board
Miss K. Lade
London County Council
*London County Council Staff Association
†Professor H. Maier
*Manchester Children's Committee
*Miss F. L. Martin
Methodist Homes for the Aged
*Mr W. H. E. Morgan
*Mr E. W. Murray
National and Local Government Officers' Association

*National Association of Approved Schools' Staffs
National Association for Mental Health
*National Association of Nursery Matrons
National Corporation for the Care of Old People
National Council for the Unmarried Mother and her Child
National Old People's Welfare Council
*National Society of Children's Nurseries
National Union of Public Employees
Northern Ireland—Association of Welfare Committees
Northern Ireland—Ministry of Education
Northern Ireland—Ministry of Health and Local Government
Northern Ireland—Ministry of Home Affairs
†Professor H. Phillips
Miss Leila Rendell
Residential Child Care Association
Royal College of Nursing and National Council of Nurses of the United Kingdom
*Salvation Army
*Scottish Approved Schools Staff Association
*Scottish Children's Officers Association
*Scottish Council for the Unmarried Mother and her Child
*Scottish Education Department
*Scottish Home and Health Department
*Scottish Society for Mentally Handicapped Children
Spastics Society
†Professor Peter Townsend
Women's Royal Voluntary Service
†Mr R. C. Wright
†Dame Eileen Younghusband

APPENDIX B

THE SURVEY QUESTIONNAIRE
AND LIST OF TABLES

I. THE QUESTIONNAIRE

(The following questionnaire is the white one we used for Children's Homes and other Homes. The other two were a blue one used for schools and other establishments employing teaching staff, and a green one for old people's Homes. All three questionnaires asked identical questions but the age-groups for residents differed and there were some differences in the qualifications we asked for. The questionnaire for Schools also asked about teaching staff and day pupils.)

RESIDENTIAL HOMES AND HOSTELS

NOTES FOR RESPONDENTS

1. This questionnaire is addressed to residential Homes or Hostels but sometimes in order to save space we use the word 'institution' to cover them.

Throughout the questionnaire we use the word 'clients' instead of inmates or residents.

'Clientèle-care staff' means all those staff concerned with looking after the clients and who are not mainly engaged in office or domestic work.

2. *Question 3*
Type of Home or Hostel. Please state the official designation or the types of people cared for, e.g. home for the mentally infirm, or mother and baby home, or in the case of a children's home, whether it caters for any special category, e.g. physically handicapped, E.S.N., and so on.

3. *Question 5*
Sponsoring Authorities. Under 5 (a) please give the name of the authority responsible for the management of the home or hostel, whether it is a local authority, a voluntary, private or religious organization.

Under 5 (b) please state whether the Government Department is the Ministry of Health, the Home Office, the Scottish Home and Health Department, or any other central government Department. If only the local authority is responsible for inspection, state 'None'.

4. *Question 6*
Total Accommodation for Clients. The replies to questions 6 (a) and (b) should exclude homeless families, but include clients in Mother and Baby

homes. In homes catering for mothers and babies or mothers and young children, please record the mother only.

For question 6 (a) please give the number of people (excluding staff) that your accommodation is designed to house, indicating their age and sex where appropriate. Where the accommodation is for clients of either sex, please use column three only.

5. *Questions 8, 9 and 10*
   (a) Replies should relate to the number of staff, including the head of the institution, on the payroll on November 30, 1963.
   (b) Part-time means less than 30 hours per week.
   (c) Where the spouse of a member of the staff is resident and does some work in the Home or Hostel, this person should be included as a part-time or full-time worker as appropriate, in the resident column.
   (d) Where Homes are attached, e.g. to a hospital, and share staff, these should be entered as part-time workers.
   (e) Students on the payroll should be included, but other students excluded.

6. *Question 20*
If there is any aspect of your institution's staffing which has not been covered by the questionnaire, please comment in the space provided.

We are particularly interested to know if the head of the institution has other duties, e.g. case work outside the home.

INSTRUCTIONS FOR COMPLETION
Questions marked * are those where you should refer to the notes before filling in the answer.

Please record answers by placing a tick

Or, where applicable, by entering a number

Or, where a written answer is required, by recording it in the space provided.
N.B. *Answers to the questions should relate to the position on November 30, 1963. The head of the Institution should be included in your replies about staff.*

PART I GENERAL

For office use only

1. Name of Home or Hostel ....

2. Address ....
   .... Tel. No......................

*3. Type of Institution (see Note 2).................................

.... ——————

4. In what year was the main part of your building constructed?

.... ——————

*5. Sponsoring authorities (see Note 3).
(a) Authority or Committee responsible for the management
of the Home or Hostel:
Name..
Address.. ——————

(b) Government department or departments, if any, responsible for inspection... ——————

*6. (a) Total accommodation for clients (see note 4. Homeless families should not be included in your reply.)

(b) Present actual numbers of clients (Do not include homeless families).

| | Accommodation | | | | | Actual numbers in Residence | |
Male	Female	Either	Total		Male	Female	Total
				Under 5 years			
				5 to 14 years			
				15 to 20 years			
				21 to 59 years			
				60 and over			
				Total			

7. Does your Home cater (in whole or in part) for home-
less families? (Mothers and babies in short stay homes   *Yes*   *No*
should be included in the reply to Question 6, and not
here.)   ....

*8. Give details of the present number of staff (see note 5).
The head of the institution should be included in 'Clientèle-care' staff.

[Q. 8. cont.]

Staff primarily engaged on	Total	Resident *in the same building as the clients or in an extension to it*		Resident *in separate accom. in the grounds or in provided accom. outside the grounds*		Non-resident	
		Full-time	*Part-time*	*Full-time*	*Part-time*	*Full-time*	*Part-time*
Clientèle-care							
Domestic work (including cooking, gardening, etc.)							
Office and Secretarial work							
Total							

*9. (*a*) How many staff vacancies are there on your establishment at present?

Staff primarily engaged on	Total	Resident *in the same building as the clients or in an extension to it*		Resident *in separate accom. in the grounds or in provided accom. outside the grounds*		Non-resident	
		Full-time	*Part-time*	*Full-time*	*Part-time*	*Full-time*	*Part-time*
Clientèle-care							
Domestic work (including cooking, gardening, etc.)							
Office and Secretarial work							
Total							

(*b*) How many of the above staff vacancies have been unfilled for more than six months?

Clientèle-care   ....

Domestic   ....

Office and Secretarial   ....

PART II   CLIENTÈLE-CARE STAFF

10. State how many of your *Clientèle-care* Staff, including the head of the institution are (see note 5):

| | Resident | | | Non-resident | |
Male	Female	Total	Male	Female	Total

Under 21 years

21 to 49 years

50 years and over

11. Of your *resident* clientèle-care staff, how many are:

Married women with *husband* working *full-time* in Home

Married women with *husband* working *part-time* in Home

Married women with *husband not* working in Home

Total

Married men with *wife* working *full-time* in Home

Married men with *wife* working *part-time* in Home

Married men with *wife not* working in Home

Total

Single women (including widows and those separated or divorced)

Single men (including widowers and those separated or divorced)

(For office use only)

12. How many of your *clientèle-care* staff, including the head of the institution, have the following qualifications? (Enter *all* the qualifications of your staff, including those with more than one qualification.)

	Full-time	Part-time	Total

S.R.N.

S.C.M.

[cont. over].

R.S.C.N.

S.E.N.

N.N.E.B.

Nursery Warden's Certificate

Certificate in the Residential Care of Children
(C.T.C. in Child Care or Scottish Advisory
Council Certificate)

Or formal training qualification awarded by a
voluntary organization

Certificate of Education (awarded for successful
completion of Training College or Institute
course)

Domestic Science Certificate or Diploma

Technical qualification for teaching of skilled
crafts, e.g. City and Guilds Certificate

University degree

University diploma or certificate in Social Science

None of the above

(For office use only)

Please state any other qualifications...
....
....

13. How many clientèle-care staff, *excluding* the head of the institution,
    have been appointed in the past twelve months?

　　(*a*) As replacements in existing posts.

	Resident		Non-resident	
	Full-time	*Part-time*	*Full-time*	*Part-time*
Men	———	———	———	———
Women	———	———	———	———
Total	———	———	———	———

(*b*) To fill newly established posts (e.g. due to expansion)?

	Resident		Non-resident	
	Full-time	Part-time	Full-time	Part-time
Men				
Women				
Total				

14. How many clientèle-care staff, *excluding* the head of the institution, have left during the past twelve months?

	Resident		Non-resident	
	Full-time	Part-time	Full-time	Part-time
Men				
Women				
Total				

15. How many clientèle-care staff, *excluding* the head of the institution, left during the last twelve months because of (enter main reason for each loss only):

	Resident				Non-resident			
	Full-time		Part-time		Full-time		Part-time	
	M	F	M	F	M	F	M	F
Marriage/maternity								
Leaving profession								
Moving to a similar post in another Home or Hostel								
To obtain training								
Promotion								
Reasons unknown								
Other reasons (please state reason in space below)								

Other reasons for leaving ....
....
....
....

16. *Head of Institution* ————
How many people have held this post over the last five
years? ————
Where this is a joint (i.e. husband and wife) appointment, count husband and wife as one.

17. Would you please give your views on the accommodation provided for your resident clientèle-care staff. Please rate each aspect of such accommodation (privacy, amount of space, heating, cooking facilities, etc.) in terms of either completely satisfactory, fairly satisfactory or less than satisfactory.

(a) *Accommodation for the Head of the Institution*

	Completely satisfactory	Fairly satisfactory	Less than satisfactory
Privacy			
Space			
Heating			
Amenities Bathroom			
Lavatory			
Personal cooking facilities			
Personal laundry facilities			

(b) *Accommodation for the married members of the staff*

	Completely satisfactory	Fairly satisfactory	Less than satisfactory
Privacy			
Space			
Heating			
Amenities Bathroom			
Lavatory			
Personal cooking facilities			
Personal laundry facilities			

(c) Accommodation for the single members of the staff

	Completely satisfactory	Fairly satisfactory	Less than satisfactory
Privacy			
Space			
Heating			
Amenities Bathroom			
Lavatory			
Personal cooking facilities			
Personal laundry facilities			

(d) Accommodation for the student members of the staff

	Completely satisfactory	Fairly satisfactory	Less than satisfactory
Privacy			
Space			
Heating			
Amenities Bathroom			
Lavatory			
Personal cooking facilities			
Personal laundry facilities			

18. Do you have any of the following staff rooms:

Staff sitting room(s) for exclusive staff use   YES   NO

....

Staff sitting room(s) used for other purposes as well	YES	NO ....
Separate staff dining room	YES	NO ....
Combined dining and sitting room	YES	NO ....
Separate staff recreation room	YES	NO ....
Changing room for non-resident staff	YES	NO ....

Any other staff rooms (please state) ....
....
....

19. Is the Home within reasonable distance of shops, cinemas, dance halls and other recreational facilities for staff?

	Shops		*Cinemas, etc.*	
Within 20 minutes walk	YES	NO	YES	NO ....
On a bus route with services at least every half hour	YES	NO	YES	NO ....

*20. General remarks on the Questionnaire, if any (see note 6). Please continue overleaf if necessary.

II. QUALIFICATIONS—DESCRIPTION OF TERMS

Heads of Homes were asked to state how many of their care staff had certain qualifications. The Census Sub-Committee selected those which were relevant to the group being cared for, or which staff were likely to have. The following are the full descriptions of the qualifications we asked about:

All Homes were asked to state how many staff had:

S.R.N. = State Registered Nurse
S.E.N. = State Enrolled Nurse
Domestic Science Certificate or Diploma
University Degree
University Diploma or Certificate in Social Science
None of the above
Other qualifications. If any of these were relevant, they were tabulated as 'other qualifications', but other nursing qualifications, e.g. Royal Army Nursing Corps, Registered Fever Nurse, etc., were tabulated as nursing qualifications.

In addition *Schools* were also asked whether staff had:

R.S.C.N. = Registered Sick Children's Nurse

S.C.M. = State Certified Midwife

Certificate in the Residential Care of Children

Formal training qualification awarded by a voluntary organization = qualification awarded by one of the large voluntary organizations who had training courses before the C.T.C. courses were set up and who awarded their own certificates at that time. (When these courses were recognized by the C.T.C. their students became eligible for the Certificate in Residential Child Care.)

Certificate of Education = teacher's training certificate awarded after the successful completion of teacher's training at a Training College or Institute, or College of Education.

Technical qualifications for teaching of skilled crafts, such as carpentry, e.g. City and Guilds Certificate.

Children's Homes and other Homes were asked about all the above qualifications and in addition were asked whether staff had:

N.N.E.B. = National Nursery Examination Board
Nursery Warden's Certificate
} These are recognized qualifications for nursery nurses.

Old People's Homes. This group alone were asked how many staff had taken the 14-week training course offered by the National Old People's Welfare Council.

III. LIST OF TABLES

The following tables, giving absolute numbers and percentages, are all those we have extracted from the census returns; the tables in the text of Chapter 4 are based on them. These tables are available for consultation either at the National Council of Social Service, 26 Bedford Square, London, W.C.1, or at the National Institute for Social Work Training, Mary Ward House, Tavistock Place, London, W.C.1, or rotaprinted sets can be purchased from the National Council of Social Service.

A. OLD PEOPLE'S HOMES

All tables split by sponsoring authority and size of Home

1. Residents of Old People's Homes, split by sex, and age. Ratios of care staff to residents (Q.6).

2. Care Staff, resident and non-resident, full-time and part-time (Q. 8).

3. Total Staff vacancies and vacancies unfilled for six months. Care staff; domestic staff; office staff (Q. 9).

4. Resident and non-resident Care Staff, split by age (Q. 10).

5. Resident Care Staff split by sex, marital status and employment of spouses in the Home (Q. 11).

6. Qualifications of all care staff, full- and part-time (Q. 12).

7.   Resident and non-resident full-time care staff appointed in the preceding twelve months, to fill existing vacancies and to fill newly established posts (Q. 13).

8.   Resident and non-resident full-time care staff who left in the preceding twelve months (Q. 14).

9.   Reasons given for leaving (Q. 15).

10.   Turnover of Heads of Homes over preceding five years (Q. 16).

11.   Views of Heads of Homes on provided staff accommodation, assessed for privacy, space, heating and amenities (bathroom, lavatory, personal cooking and laundry facilities) for Heads themselves; for married staff; for single staff (Q. 17).

12.   Provision of other staff accommodation—staff sitting rooms and whether for exclusive staff use, separate dining room or combined sitting and dining room, staff recreation room, changing room for non-resident staff (Q. 18).

13.   Isolation of Home (Q. 19): whether Home within 20 minutes walk of shops, cinemas and other recreation; whether Home on bus route with half-hourly service to shops, cinemas, etc.

B.   CHILDREN'S HOMES

All tables split by sponsoring authority and size of Home

1.   Children in Homes, divided by age and sex. Ratio of children to care staff.

2.   Care staff, resident and non-resident, full- and part-time (Q. 8).

3.   Total staff vacancies and vacancies unfilled for six months. Care staff; domestic staff; office staff (Q. 9).

4.   Resident and non-resident care staff, split by age (Q. 10).

5.   Resident care staff, split by sex, marital status and employment of spouses in the Home (Q. 11).

6.   Qualifications of all care staff, full-time and part-time (Q. 12).

7.   Resident and non-resident full-time care staff appointed in the preceding twelve months to fill existing vacancies and to fill newly established posts (Q. 13).

8.   Resident and non-resident full-time care staff who left in preceding twelve months (Q. 14).

9.   Reasons given for leaving (Q. 15).

10.   Turnover of heads of Homes over preceding five years (Q. 16).

11.   Views of Heads of Homes on provided staff accommodation, assessed for privacy, space, heating and amenities (bathroom, lavatory, personal cooking and laundry facilities) for Heads themselves; for married staff; for single staff; for students (Q. 17).

12.   Provision of other staff accommodation—staff sitting rooms and whether for exclusive staff use, separate dining room or combined sitting and dining room, staff recreation room, changing room for non-resident staff (Q. 18).

13. Isolation of Home (Q. 19): whether Home within 20 minutes walk of shops, cinemas and other recreation; whether Home on bus route with half-hourly service to shops, cinemas, etc.

C. OTHER HOMES:

Reception Homes, Hostels for working boys and girls, Nurseries for under-fives, Mother and Baby Homes, Homes for physically handicapped adults, Homes for mentally ill and mentally handicapped adults.
All tables split by type of Home only.

1. Summary Table of Residents, split by sex and age. Ratio of Care Staff to Residents (Q. 6).
2. Care staff, resident and non-resident, full-time and part-time (Q. 8).
3. Total staff vacancies and vacancies unfilled for six months. Care staff; domestic staff; office staff (Q. 9).
4. Resident and non-resident care staff, split by age (Q. 10).
5. Resident care staff, split by sex, marital status and employment of spouses in the Home (Q. 11).
6. Qualifications of all care staff, full-time and part-time (Q. 12).
7. Resident and non-resident full-time care staff appointed in the preceding twelve months to fill existing vacancies and to fill newly established posts (Q. 13).
8. Resident and non-resident full-time care staff who left in the preceding twelve months (Q. 14).
9. Reasons given for leaving (Q. 15).
10. Turnover of Heads of Homes over preceding five years (Q. 16).
11. Views of Heads of Homes on provided staff accommodation, assessed for privacy, space, heating and amenities (bathroom, lavatory, personal cooking and laundry facilities) for Heads themselves; for married staff; for single staff; for students (Q. 17).
12. Provision of other staff accommodation—staff sitting rooms and whether for exclusive staff use, separate dining room or combined sitting and dining room, staff recreation room, changing room for non-resident staff (Q. 18).
13. Isolation of Home (Q. 19): whether Home within 20 minutes walk of shops, cinemas and other recreations; whether Home on bus route with half-hourly service to shops, cinemas, etc.

D. APPROVED SCHOOLS, REMAND HOMES AND SPECIAL SCHOOLS
All tables split by three types of approved school, by remand Homes and by six types of special school.

1. Summary Table of Residents, split by sex and age. Ratio of care staff to residents (Q. 6).
2. Care staff, resident and non-resident, full-time and part-time. Total teaching staff (Q. 8).
3. Total staff vacancies and vacancies unfilled for six months. Care staff; teaching staff; domestic staff; office staff (Q. 9).

4. Resident and non-resident staff, split by age (Q. 10).

5. Resident care staff, split by sex, marital status and employment of spouses in the Home (Q. 11).

6. Qualifications of all care staff, full- and part-time (Q. 12).

7. Resident and non-resident full-time care staff appointed in preceding twelve months, to fill existing vacancies and newly established posts (Q. 13).

8. Resident and non-resident full-time care staff who left in the preceding twelve months (Q. 14).

9. Reasons given for leaving (Q. 15).

10. Turnover of Heads of Homes over preceding five years (Q. 16).

11. Views of Heads of Homes on provided staff accommodation, assessed for privacy, space, heating and amenities (bathroom, lavatory, personal cooking and laundry facilities) for Heads themselves; for married staff; for single staff; for students (Q. 17).

12. Provision of other staff accommodation—staff sitting rooms and whether for exclusive staff use, separate dining room or combined sitting and dining room, staff recreation room, changing room for non-resident staff (Q. 18).

13. Isolation of Home (Q. 19): whether Home within 20 minutes walk of shops, cinemas and other recreation; whether Home on bus route with half-hourly service to shops, cinemas, etc.

APPENDIX C

OUTLINE OF A TWO YEAR TRAINING COURSE

1. The Committee were hesitant about putting forward for publication their outline of a Course for Residential Care. Once material is in print it tends to assume an authority far greater than is warranted. This outline is offered not as a blueprint, but rather as a basis for discussion. Apart from the 'Outline for a basic course of training for residential work with children and young people' issued by the Central Training Council in Child Care—for which we make grateful acknowledgment—not only had we little on which to build, but we have been unable even to try out our suggested outline, and so inevitably it comes unrehearsed. Doubtless it says too much on the one hand and too little on the other; it is too detailed and not detailed enough. But the load of teaching has been assessed and we are convinced that some such syllabus would work within the two years we have recommended and cover the needs of the many types of staff with whom we have been concerned.

2. Any outline offered at this stage may be superseded by one devised by the proposed national training body after one or two year's experience. We have not matched it with any suggestions for the proposed One Year specialized courses; but the outline for the basic course of the Central Training Council in Child Care should prove a useful comparison here, and it would be possible, though at considerable loss, to extract the special content for each of the different fields from the course that is set out on subsequent pages, and use this as an outline for the One Year courses.

3. It would have been tempting to include other specialisms than the four suggested, but this would have led to a fragmentation of the course and the common content would have been dissipated. We selected the main groups in residential care on which to focus the training, and we believe that the course as outlined will meet the needs of the great majority in the work. The needs of some groups may have to be further developed in particular courses and balances may need to be redressed. There are sizeable groups, for example children in special schools and homes, to meet whose needs it would seem that staff should study in the special fields of children and the physically handicapped. The taking of these two special subjects in full might, however, amount to too heavy a load and the programmes of such students would need to be designed with this point in mind; it might well be that they would not attend all the classes dealing with the handicaps of adults.

4. We have not suggested the level of teaching of the subjects included. We are aware that the detailing of the course may give the impression of greater complexity and higher intellectual demands than we intend. It is assumed that subjects will be taught in a practical way, that students will not be required to have specific academic qualifications and that the most natural

setting would be a non-university centre of adult education. It must not be forgotten that once interest is aroused, and especially with the use of new educational methods, students are capable of study at a much greater depth and intensity than many of them have shown in a previous educational setting which did not extend or stimulate them.

SELECTION OF STUDENTS

5. Careful selection of individual students will be important, as the twenty years' experience of the Central Training Council in Child Care has shown. It will clearly be of great advantage if students have had prior experience of residential work before embarking on the two-year course, but this should not be a rigid requirement. Although no specific educational qualification will be demanded, course tutors will need to be satisfied that intending students will be able to meet the considerable demands of the course. It is assumed that only those students who show promise of sufficient maturity and personal suitability for residential work will be selected. For some people residential work holds no appeal, but others who may be quite unsuitable are attracted all too easily. The help of the national training body will doubtless be very valuable in maintaining comparable standards in selection.

LENGTH AND GENERAL DESIGN

6. The Course is designed for a period of twenty-four months, allowing for six weeks holiday in each year. It is suggested that between nine and ten months should be given to learning by means of supervised practical experience. Part of this practical work might be undertaken concurrently with study and part for full-time periods, and there should be room for experiment in pattern and sequence. Experience suggests, however, that one period of practical work—normally in the field of the special interest of the student—should extend over a period of two to three months in one residential setting; that this should take place at some stage after the first year of the course; that another period should be spent in a different type of institution, and that some experience should be arranged in a social service related to families or individuals not in residence.

7. Initial study should not be prolonged for more than two months without experience of practical work. Sufficient time should be given throughout the course and particularly at the end, to draw together material and experience from both methods of learning.

8. Close relation between study and practical work is essential and for this reason there should be regular consultation with the staff who supervise the students' practical work so that they will be closely identified with the training as a whole. The partnership of tutors and supervisors should be sustained throughout the course by regular staff meetings, consultations about the progress of individual students and reviews of the content and methods of training.

9. The programme of study should be designed so that, in addition to lectures, provision is made for seminars in small groups and each student

should have regular tutorial discussion and time to undertake an individual project on the line of his particular interest.

10. The tutorials and seminars in the second year of the course would be centred on principles and practice in the chosen field of study and especially directed at defining the nature of the task and the role of the worker in this field. In the tutorials there will be an opportunity to show how the other courses feed in, for example, to the basic subject of home-making.

11. A suitable plan might provide each year for three terms of study in the training centre of about nine weeks each. During the first year the content of study common to all types of residential work would be undertaken by all students. At the same time some seminar discussions would be provided on the subject of the student's special choice and the proportion of time given to these special subjects would be increased during the second year.

12. Some suggestions are made below as to the time to be given to each particular subject. The balance will be the responsibility of those planning the particular courses, and it may well be that this will vary from time to time according to the availability of lecturers and to any particular emphases that the courses develop.

13. We would urge that one day a week should be free of lectures and used for reading, tutorials, seminars, visits, etc., and that there should not be more than three sessions on any one day, a 'session' being a lecture and discussion for an hour and a half. The weighting has been so arranged as to work out at about seven sessions a week, and never more than ten. The amount of time devoted to each course, as indicated below, fits in with such a time table even if a student takes two special choice subjects in his second year.

ASSESSMENT OF STUDENTS

14. We are aware of the trends and fashions in this matter and there is probably no justification for dogmatism on this point. We are persuaded that assessment of a student's progress should be a continuing process. At the end of the course the student's whole record, his written and practical work, his contribution to seminars and in tutorials and his individual project should be taken into account rather than an assessment based solely on written or oral examination. Some would urge the need for a 'testing' situation, albeit freed from the trammels of a time limit; others would emphasize the practical situation into which the student will move and the differing strains that this imposes from those of class room or the blank page.

15. Here again the guidance of the national training body will be indispensible especially as it will need to maintain a comparable standard of achievement as between the various courses.

PLAN FOR A TWO YEAR COURSE

Common Content Subjects:
(1) Home Making and Household Management.
    (Once weekly throughout the first year.)

(2) Human Growth and Behaviour.
  (Twice weekly throughout first four terms.)
(3) Health.
  (Once weekly for two terms in first year.)
(4) Social Relationships.
  (Once weekly throughout first four terms.)
(5) Individual and Social Interests and Activities.
  (Once weekly throughout first year.)
(6) Social Services.
  (Once weekly throughout first year.)
(7) Ethical and Religious Issues.
  (Once weekly for the last two terms of the first year.)

Special Choice Subjects
A. Children and young people.
B. Elderly.
C. Physically handicapped of all ages, including the blind and the deaf.
D. Socially handicapped (with special reference to the mentally disordered
   and the socially maladjusted).
  Each of the Special Choice Subjects will be pursued under the following
headings:
  (8) Special needs and problems.
    (Once weekly throughout the second year.)
  (9) Health.
    (Once weekly for two terms in the second year.)
(10) Residential Communities.
    (Once weekly for two terms in the second year.)
(11) Social Services.
    (Once weekly throughout second year.)

CONTENT OF COMMON SUBJECTS

1. *Home Making and Household Management*
16. The nature and variety of residential communities. Administration.
Staff responsibilities and relationships. Provision of comfortable and attractive homes for residents and staff. Rooms, furnishing, equipment, maintenance, budgeting, food values, catering. Planned use of time, labour,
money and materials.

2. *Human Growth and Behaviour*
17. Normal development and individual needs from early infancy, through
adolescence to old age. Physical, emotional, social and intellectual aspects:
their inter-relation. Heredity and environment. Individual differences.
Development of personality: motivation, conscious and unconscious. Significance of family relationships at all ages. Adjustment and maladjustment.
Behaviour problems associated with deprivation, handicap and stress.

3. Health

18. Stages and variations in physical growth from infancy to old age. Good health, its influence on attitudes and behaviour. Diet, physical conditions. Physical handicaps. Emotional disturbance. Psychosomatic disorder. Use of medical services: the general practitioner, school health service, hospitals. Home nursing. Care in infection and illness. First Aid.

4. Social Relationships

19. Group relations. Advantages and limitations of living in a residential group: opportunities and frustrations: significance for individuals. Acceptance and rejection. Network of relationships: staff, residents and their families. Contrast with family life. Effect of separation. Maintenance of contacts. Compensations. Meaning of a therapeutic community. Planning for order with individual freedom. Relation of residential community to neighbourhood.

5. Individual and Social Interests and Activities

20. Cultivation of special interests. Group activities, planned and unplanned. Town and country pleasures. Enjoyment of the arts. Appraisal of modern methods of communication and entertainment. Hobbies, pets and gardens. Neighbourhood provisions for enjoyment and involvement.

6. Social Services

21. Statutory and voluntary services designed to meet the needs of the individual, family and community. The social scene in Britain. Central and local government. Voluntary organizations. Committee responsibilities. Recent trends and developments with special reference to domiciliary services, community care and the changing functions of residential institutions. Team approach to distress and need: co-operation with other workers in the social services. Office organization. Records and correspondence.

7. Ethical and Religious Issues

22. [Note: *These issues have a particular significance in residential settings, where staff of differing views may share responsibility for people of divers beliefs, race and background. They are especially relevant to some groups, e.g. children and old people. Because the staff of children's homes inevitably influence the whole upbringing of the many children in their care, attention is drawn to the further note in the section of the syllabus dealing with children, paragraphs 31 and 32 below.*]

23. Introduction to ethical and religious concepts applicable to various cultural backgrounds. The relationship between personal conviction and respect for the beliefs of others. Criteria for making judgments and decisions. The respective claims of the individual and the group. Theories of punishment. Problems associated with pain and death. The application of general principles, e.g. honesty, fairness, acceptance, in particular group settings.

Special Choice Subjects

A. CHILDREN AND YOUNG PEOPLE

[Note: *The following outline is intended for students who expect to work with children of any age, some of whom will be with their mothers in mother and baby homes or rehabilitation centres. Each phase of development can only properly be understood by reference to the continuum of physical and mental growth. Nevertheless, the care of adolescents in residential settings, of children who are handicapped, and of babies and very young children will call for additional study and specially chosen experience. The syllabus for these additional studies, which presumably would include lectures, seminars and tutorials, is not suggested here. It might be that certain Centres would include a detailed study of one of these groups as the recognized emphasis of the Course, but this should not militate against the concept of children's development as a continuing and integrated process.*]

8. Special Needs and Problems

25. Physical, intellectual, emotional and social development at all ages. Individual differences. Problems arising from disabilities in intelligence and emotion and from physical handicaps. Significance of maternal, paternal and family relationships at all ages. Relationships with other adults. Deprivation. Adjustment and maladjustment. Meeting of children's needs at different levels through play, activity, involvement, etc. Peer groups. Problems characteristic of different ages. The transition from the residential Home to the ordinary world.

9. Health

26. Environmental requirements. Factors making for good health. Interrelation of physical with other aspects of development. Symptoms of stress and ill-health. Common illnesses and disorders. Recognition of the need for medical care. Home nursing and first aid. Health records. Precaution against and control of infection. Personal hygiene. Special problems of handicapped and backward children. Prevention of accidents. Suitable and attractive meals.

10. Residential Communities

27. Purpose and aims of different types of residential communities. Merits and limitations of various sizes and groupings. Motives and attitudes of staff. Balance of individual care and group living. Provision for individual privacy and interests. Reception and preparation for change of placement or leaving. Contact with relatives, friends and the wider community.

28. Methods of encouraging responsibility and independence. Rules, routine, rewards and sanctions in different types of Homes and schools.

29. Assessing individual progress, staff discussion, records. Co-operation with teachers, social workers, doctors. Statutory regulations.

11. Social Services

30. Main statutory and voluntary education, health and social services for

children and young people. Recent history and present trends. Education departments, day schools and related services, boarding special schools. Children's departments: reception into care, adoption, fostering, children's Homes. Approved schools, remand Homes. Maternity and child health services. Provision for unmarried mothers and their children. Day nurseries and nursery schools and related services. Provisions for physical and mental health, e.g. child guidance clinics. Hospital care. Reasons for residence in cases of maladjustment, subnormality or delinquency. Juvenile courts: their constitution, powers and related services.

Note on Ethical and Religious Issues

31. *The upbringing of children must involve responsibility for their developing sense of moral values. Adults who care for them cannot contract out of the effect of their own attitudes. There is also a legal obligation to ensure that children are brought up in the religious faith of their parents.*

32. *Students who will be responsible for young people will need to clarify their own views and to be aware and tolerant of different individual beliefs. They should know enough about the various religious faiths to which children belong to respect their observances and to encourage the personal help of ministers of religion. Students may also want guidance about provision to be made for communal worship or other observances and about special Sunday activities in Homes.*

B. THE ELDERLY

8. Special Needs and Problems

33. Physical and psychological characteristics of the ageing process and of being old and infirm. The relevance and irrelevance of chronological age. Interpretation of the attitudes of old to young and young to old. The significance of the continuing role of the family.

34. Variety of needs according to the nature and degree of dependence of the able-bodied elderly. Those needing 'care and attention'. The handicapped. The physically and mentally infirm. The dying.

9. Health

35. Appropriate physical care. Warmth. Suitable and attractive meals. Encouragement of independence, e.g. in dressing and bathing. Value of a flexible regime and individual provision of, e.g. chairs, bed-rests and other aids. Common infirmities and disorders and the extent to which these are susceptible to treatment, e.g. strokes, mental confusion, incontinence, behaviour disorders. Common accidents and dangers and their prevention. Care of drugs. Special needs in terminal illness, death and last offices.

36. The role of hospitals, psycho-geriatric clinics, geriatric consultants, general practitioners, local health authorities, trained nurses.

10. Residential Communities

37. Characteristics of different residential settings, e.g. sheltered housing, long-stay hospital units. Design and siting of Homes: special provisions,

e.g. ramps, rails, good lighting. Acceptable care, avoidance of institutionalization and isolation. Special aspects of the group situation. Role and relationships of staff. Sharing responsibility between staff and residents.

11. *Social Services*
38. Old people in modern society. Pattern of family care. Role of the local authority health and welfare departments. Social security services, Housing Departments, voluntary agencies. Community services for old people in residential care. Mobilizing community interest.

C. THE PHYSICALLY HANDICAPPED OF ALL AGES (including the blind and deaf)
39. [Note: *To some extent students are more likely to have, or to develop, special interest in one or more particular class of handicap. Their interest should be reflected by guided studies and by the residential units chosen for their practical work placements. Some additional placements with field workers would be important, particularly in relation to the blind and deaf.*
40. *Although the teaching of special skills like Braille, Moon, finger spelling and signing, craft teaching, etc., would not form part of the course, students who wished to do so should be encouraged to start on such studies and practice wherever facilities were available.*]

8. *Special Needs and Problems*
41. The types of handicap, e.g. blind, partially sighted, deaf: severe physical handicaps due to congenital or other causes. Special characteristics of each group in terms of physical and social limitations and psychological implications. Multiple handicaps.
42. Changes in attitude to handicaps by society and handicapped persons themselves, from protection and dependence to self help and independence within the limit of the handicap.

9. *Health*
43. Medical aspects of various handicaps. Expectations of stabilization or deterioration. Special features of care. Role of hospitals, consultant services, rehabilitation units, general practitioners, nurses, local health authorities.
44. Practical issues; use of aids and appliances, their supervision and upkeep. Care of drugs.

10. *Residential Communities*
45. The place of residential care and the contra-indications in relation to particular handicaps. Provision for specialized or mixed groups, in terms of sex, age and type of handicap. Appropriate buildings and interior planning for promoting mobility and personal independence. Features of significance for particular groups, e.g. wide doors for wheel chairs, visual aids for the deaf. Common accidents, dangers and their prevention. The role of staff and residents.

11.   Social Services

46.   Role of the Local Authority Health and Welfare departments. Stage of development in services for the welfare of the handicapped living in their own homes. Availability of specialized staff. Contribution of the voluntary services. Liaison with the outside community for employment: recreation, religious observance, holidays, community involvement. Voluntary work by residents. The Ministry of Social Security, the Ministry of Labour services, workshops, employment of the disabled.

D. THE SOCIALLY HANDICAPPED

(With special reference to the mentally disordered and the socially maladjusted.)

47.   [Note: *There are considerable differences between the groups in this subject; students will not wish to work with the whole range of people included here. Nevertheless, it would be useful and valuable for them to know something about the needs and problems of such other groups in addition to those with whom they intend to work.*]

8.   Special Needs and Problems

48.   Types of abnormal development: subnormal and severely sub-normal children and adults. Types of mental ill health; psychosis, neurosis, addiction, psychopathy, behaviour disorders, mental deterioration in old age. Special characteristics of these groups and varieties of support needed. Degrees of responsibility. Dependence and independence. Attitudes of society towards mental disorder and social inadequacy.

9.   Health

49.   Changing concepts and methods of treatment: treatment by drugs, individual psychotherapy and treatment in groups. Dealing with psychiatric emergencies in the Home. The role of the consultant psychiatrist and general practitioner. Responsibility for medication and drugs, special diets and appliances. Special health risks for subnormal patients. Mixed mental and physical disabilities.

10.   Residential Communities

50.   Merits of residential or community care. Therapeutic communities. Different provisions needed for special groups. Interdependence of domiciliary and residential care. Acceptance of the Home or hostel as part of the community. Possibilities of employment for certain residents. Contacts with employers. Problems of living with such groups. Need for steady and stable relationships. Group counselling. Acceptance, tolerance, support, willingness to try again after failure. Factors to be considered when residents want to leave. Relationships with those who have left.

11.   Social Services

51.   Relevant legislation, e.g. the Mental Health Act. Special conditions of

employment and insurance. Psychiatric hospitals. Health and Welfare Departments of the local authorities. Youth Employment and Disablement Resettlement Officers. Probation Service and the Courts. Training Centres. Industrial Therapy organizations and sheltered workshops. Voluntary bodies, e.g. parent groups, organizations such as Alcoholics Anonymous and Samaritans, societies for helping discharged prisoners, the National Association for Mental Health.

INDEX

(figures refer to chapter and paragraph numbers)